Fauzia Khalifa Musbah

Easy Clinical Trichoscopic Approach

Fauzia Khalifa Musbah

Easy Clinical Trichoscopic Approach

LAP LAMBERT Academic Publishing

Imprint
Any brand names and product names mentioned in this book are subject to trademark, brand or patent protection and are trademarks or registered trademarks of their respective holders. The use of brand names, product names, common names, trade names, product descriptions etc. even without a particular marking in this work is in no way to be construed to mean that such names may be regarded as unrestricted in respect of trademark and brand protection legislation and could thus be used by anyone.

Cover image: www.ingimage.com

Publisher:
LAP LAMBERT Academic Publishing
is a trademark of
Dodo Books Indian Ocean Ltd. and OmniScriptum S.R.L publishing group

120 High Road, East Finchley, London, N2 9ED, United Kingdom
Str. Armeneasca 28/1, office 1, Chisinau MD-2012, Republic of Moldova, Europe
Managing Directors: Ieva Konstantinova, Victoria Ursu
info@omniscriptum.com

Printed at: see last page
ISBN: 978-620-8-11973-7

Dr. Fauzia Khalia Musbah, MD

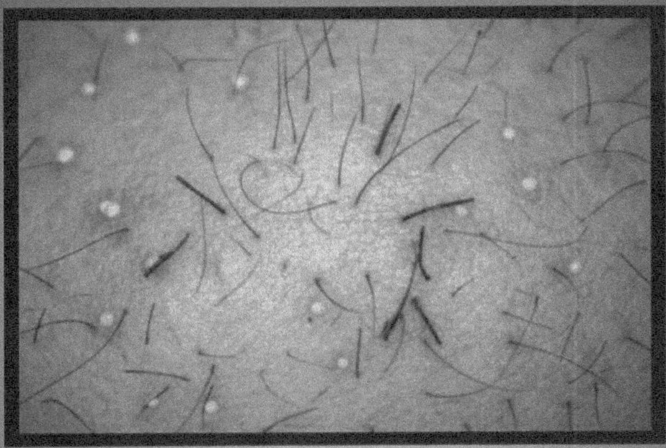

EASY CLINICAL TRICHOSCOPIC APPROACH

A PRACTICAL GUIDE TO HAIR AND SCALP DISORDERS.

First edition I 2024

Editor:

Fauzia Khalifa Musbah, MD
Assistant Professor at the Department of Dermatology
Tripoli Central Hospital

Acknowledgements

This guide has been compiled to enhance the structured, step-by-step practice of trichoscopy. The information and photographs in this book are based on clinical cases in a way that helps to learn the basics and thus forms a strong foundation for advancing to more complex learning.

Table of Contents

Hair and Scalp Dermoscopy

Dermoscopy is a diagnostic tool that magnifies the subtle clinical surface features of the scalp skin and hair abnormalities that are not visible with a standard magnifying lens.

The terms **dermoscopy** and **trichoscopy** are often used interchangeably in practice for hair and scalp examination.

I - Instruments for Scalp Dermoscopy

Trichoscopy uses **epiluminescence microscopy (ELM)** with the following types:

- Hand-held oil immersion dermoscope
- Non-polarized contact dermoscope from Heine and Welch Allyn
- Polarized and non-polarized dermatoscope - 3Gen DermLite
- Magnetic connect 40.5mm for Nikon 1 and Sony Alpha 5000
- FotoFinder video dermatoscopy

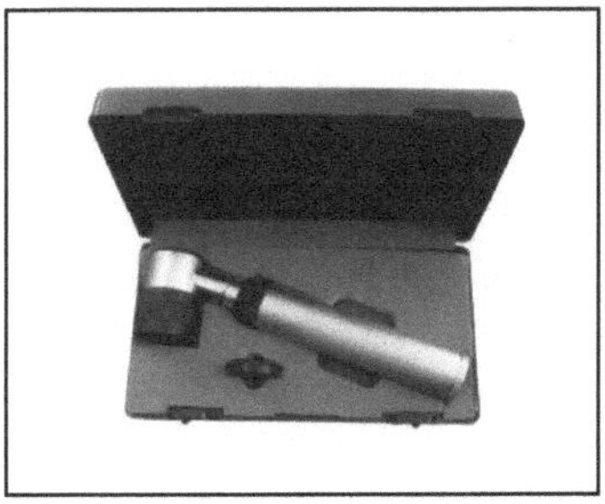

Figure 3Hand-held oil immersion dermoscope

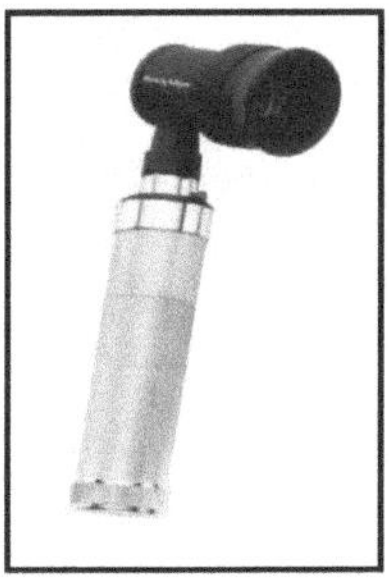

Figure 2 Non-polarized contact dermoscope from Heine and Welch Allyn

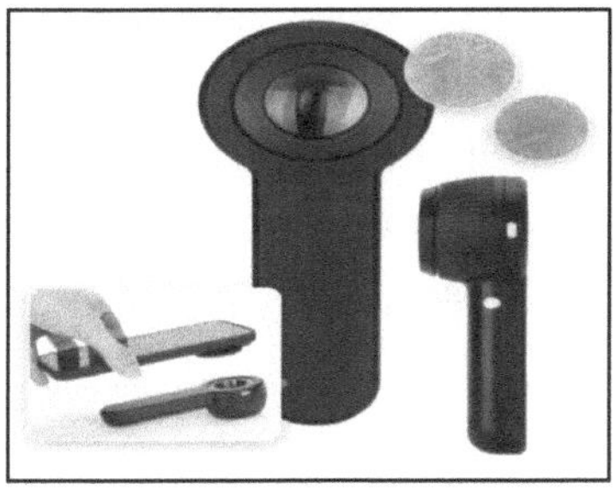

Figure 1 Polarized and non-polarized dermatoscope - 3Gen DermLite

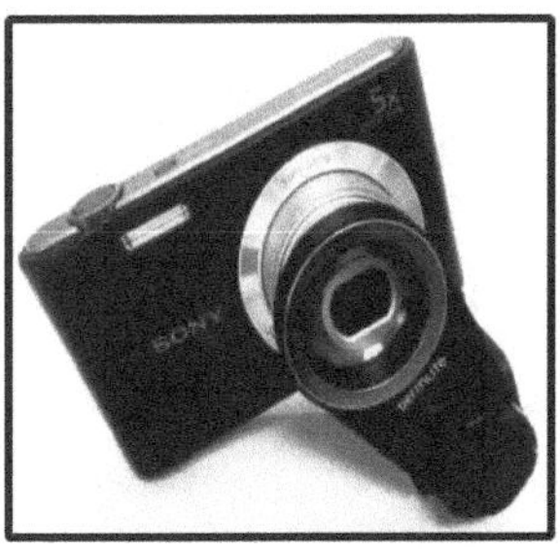

Figure 5 Magnetic connect 40.5mm for Nikon 1 and Sony Alpha 5000

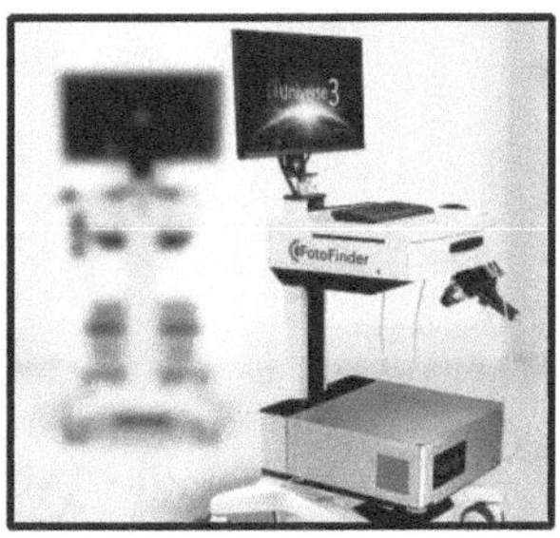

Figure 4 FotoFinder video dermatoscopy

Principles of Trichoscopy

The basic principle of trichoscopy is the illumination of the lesion with different light sources and studying it with a high-magnification lens that may or may not be connected to a camera and computer.

Components of Trichoscopy

1. **Achromatic lens:** Magnification power of 10x, 20x, and high magnification up to 1000x can be achieved in videodermoscopy.
2. **Built-in illumination system:** For better visualization of skin and hair, the use of polarized and non-polarized light sources:
   - Halogen lamps (yellow light) are placed within the handled piece
   - Light-emitting diodes (LEDs): Provide white light and have the advantage of consuming 70% less power than halogen lamps

Polarized light allows for deeper penetration and better visualization without requiring contact plates or linkage fluid. In contrast, non-polarized light penetrates more superficially.

3. **Power supply:** Hand-held instruments are usually powered by batteries and may have rechargeable handles.
4. **Built-in photography system: An** attached digital camera is needed to record and store the images.
5. **Contact plate:** Made of multi-coated silicone glass and available in different types.

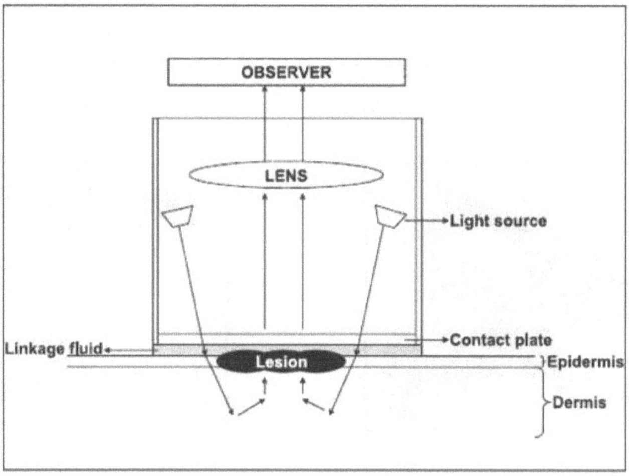

Figure 6 Optics of dermoscope.

Optical Principles

The refracted light transilluminates the lesion while passing through it and is perceived as a distinct pattern. Any light incident on skin and hair undergoes various proportions depending on the physical properties of the skin:

- Reflection
- Refraction
- Diffraction
- Absorption

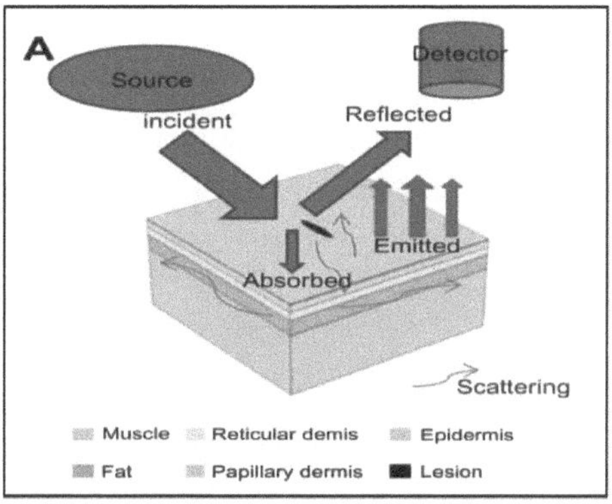

Figure 6 interaction of radiation with tissue (absorption, reflection), radiation source, and detector

Light Interaction with Tissue

- Light incident on dry, scaly skin is reflected.
- Light is reflected because the stratum corneum has a higher refractive index than 1.55 compared to 1.00 for air.
- Most of the light incident on the skin surface is reflected when visualized with a magnifying lens.
- Light incident on smooth skin allows light to pass through it, reaching the deeper dermis with less reflectance by using cross-polarization/fluid immersion; surface reflections are eliminated, rendering the cornified layer translucent.

Cross-Polarization

To achieve cross-polarization, two polarizers are needed: the source polarized filter for the light being emitted, and the polarized detector filter, which filters the light just prior to entering the lens. When the source and detector filters are perpendicular to each other, this is referred to as cross-polarization. With cross-polarization, light reflected from the stratum corneum is unable to pass through the detector filter. As a result, cross-polarization serves to eliminate light glare.

Non-polarized Light Dermoscopy	Polarized Dermoscopy
Visualizing superficial layers of the skin, such as comedo-like openings in seborrheic keratosis	Better visualization of deeper structures located at the dermoepidermal junction or superficial dermis, such as collagen and vessels

Table 1 Non-polarized Vs Polarized Dermoscopy

Linkage Fluids Used to Improve Skin Translucency

- **Immersion oil:** Causes many bubbles, making visualization difficult. It is contraindicated because it contains chlorinated paraffin and dibutyl phthalate, which have teratogenic and carcinogenic effects.
- **Olive oil**
- **Mineral oil**
- **Water:** Causes fewer bubbles but evaporates quickly, hence less preferable than oils. Besides, their refractive index is close to that of skin; hence, subsurface features may not be well seen.
- **Alcohol 70%:** Gives a better view because it eliminates air bubbles and decreases infection transmission.
- **Glycerin and gels**

Advanced Techniques

Phototrichogram: Saitoh introduced the phototrichogram in 1970. It is an automated phototrichogram in which digital image analysis is connected to a smartphone or computer. Their software measures hair quantity and quality and determines hair length, width, and current hair cycle phase.

Videotrichoscopy: This is a modification of the phototrichogram technique that can be done by either a contact or non-contact technique. Phototrichogram and TrichoScan are used to take photos as an initial step for hair investigations and hair growth, measuring the effect of therapies. It also permits visualization of hair shafts at higher magnification (about 70x and 100x).
Some of the observations have diagnostic value even where biopsy does not offer reliable differentiation, which helps in decision-making or assessing prognosis.

Note: In this book, trichoscopic examination was performed using a DL3 dermoscope (DermLite, 3Gen LLC, San Juan Capistrano, CA, USA), and trichoscopy with a 5-megapixel digital camera was attached to save the images (Magnification x10). Trichoscopic features were observed, and photographs were taken with the help of a mobile device camera.

Special Considerations

- It is better to avoid hair washing 2-3 days before trichoscopic examination because washing may eliminate important physical signs.
- Objects on the scalp that may hinder diagnosis include dirt in children, hair dye, makeup, foundation, cosmetic hair fibers, and textile fibers.
- Removing the scaly coating layer improves visibility of the blood vessels.
- Eyebrows and eyelashes are best inspected with a non-contact dermoscope. Never use alcoholic immersion fluid for eyebrows and eyelashes.
- Ultraviolet-enhanced trichoscopy (UVET) may facilitate the diagnosis of diseases that exhibit fluorescence under Wood's light.

Normal Scalp
Follicular Unit Anatomy

A single hair shaft is made of three parts:

- Medulla
- Cortex
- Cuticle

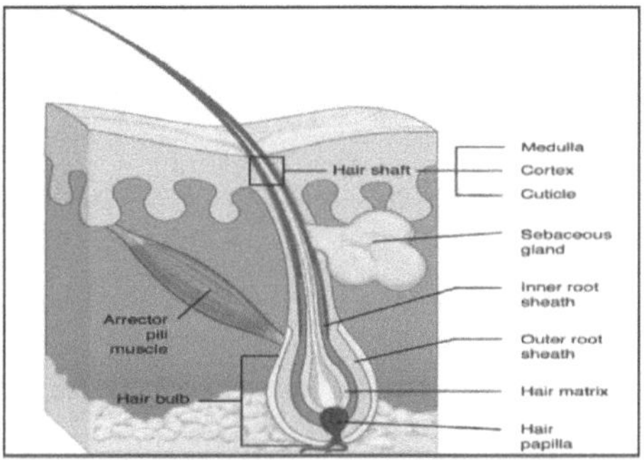

Figure 7 Hair follicles originate in the epidermis and have many different parts (Lumen, Biology for Majors).

Trichoscopic Structures and Patterns

The following need to be observed:

- Hair shafts
- Interfollicular, perifollicular space, and follicular openings: assessed for the presence of dots of different colors, pinpoint white dots corresponding to eccrine gland openings
- Pigmentary pattern
- Vascular pattern

In Normal Scalp:

- Follicular unit: 1-4 terminal hairs
- 1mm between each follicle
- Vellus hair: 1-2
- Up to 10% of the normal scalp consists of vellus hairs
- Scalp pigmentation network
- White and red dots

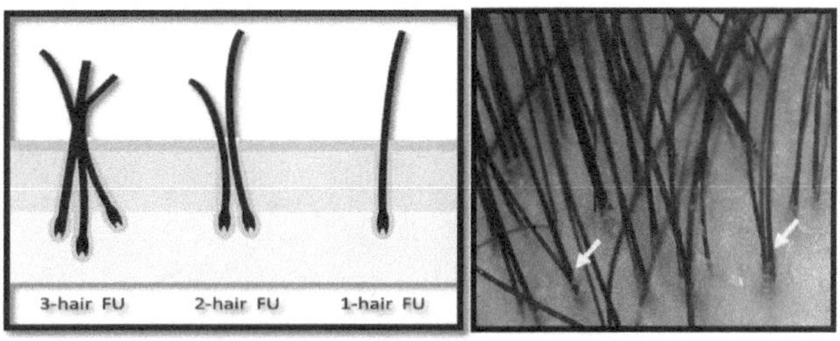

Figure 8 The number of hairs in a follicular unit varies from c to three in healthy persons.

White Scalp:

- Hair follicular unit: 2-4 terminal hairs emerge and 1-2 vellus hairs
- Interfollicular blood vessels (loop, arborizing)
- The number of hair units is less in the frontal and temporal areas than in the occipital area

Black Scalp:

- Tiny pinpoint white dots correspond to acrosyringeal and follicular openings
- Interfollicular honeycomb-like pigment network
- Hairs mostly emerge in groups

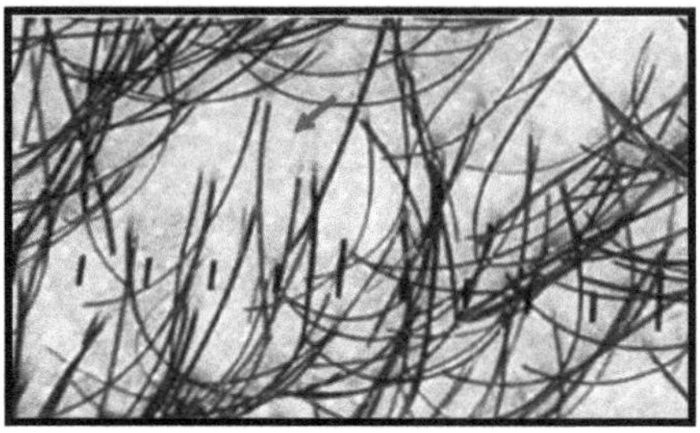

Figure 9 Tiny pinpoint white dots

Vascular Interfollicular Pattern:

Simple red linear loops: Normal scalp and most inflammatory conditions appear as multiple regularly spaced hairpin-like structures

- **Twisted (coiled) red loops:** Conditions characterized by acanthosis (psoriasis)
- **Arborizing red lines:** Tree-like pattern seen in seborrheic dermatitis

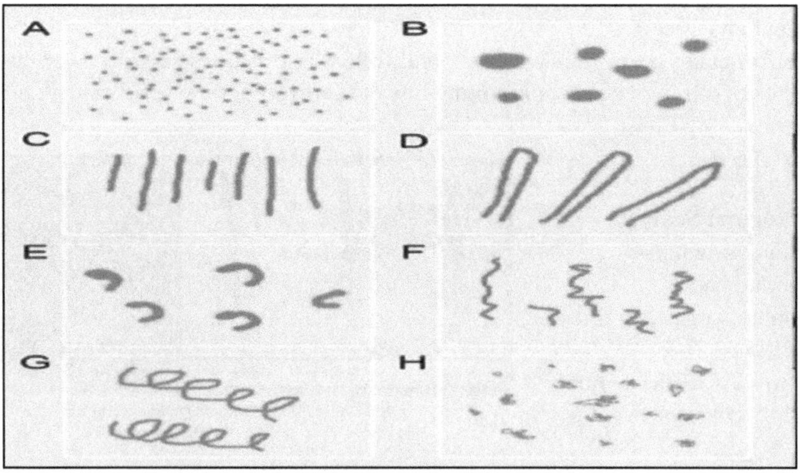

Figure 10 Vascular patterns: Vessels as dots (A), clots (B), and linear vessels (C to H). Different types of linear vessels: Straight (C); loop (D), curved; serpentine (F), helical (G), and coiled (H).

II- Trichoscopy for Hair Loss

1. Non-Scarring Alopecia: Trichoscopic Findings

1.1 Alopecia Areata

Alopecia Areata (AA) is an immune-mediated condition affecting the scalp and other hair-bearing areas of the body. AA is usually diagnosed clinically, but in cases where diagnosis is not straightforward, a biopsy is an invasive method. Instead, dermoscopy has certain findings according to the disease activity and severity, such as exclamation marks, black dots, tapered hairs, and broken hairs, which correlate with disease activity, while the presence of yellow dots and vellus hair indicates chronicity and severity of the disease.

Alopecia Areata (AA)	Alopecia Areata Totalis (AAT)	Alopecia Areata Universalis (AAU)	Alopecia Areata Ophiasis (AAO)
Solitary, rounded/oval single or multiple areas of hair loss 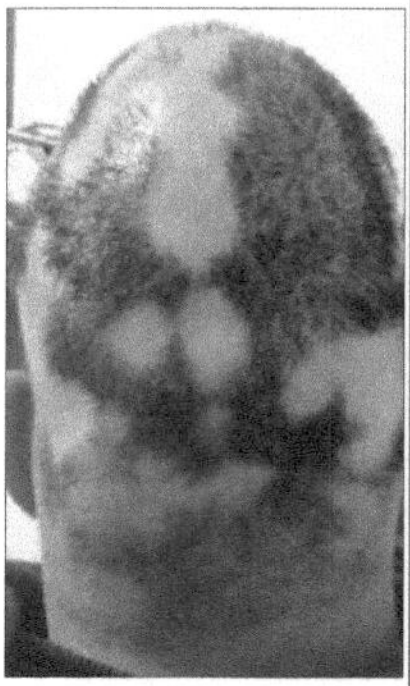	Total loss of terminal scalp hair 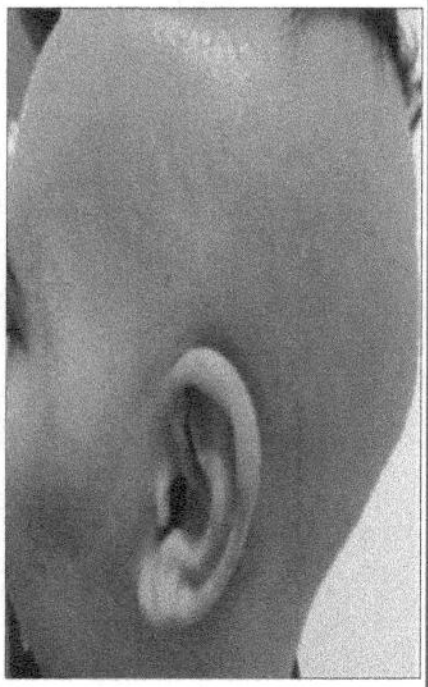	Total loss of terminal scalp and body hair 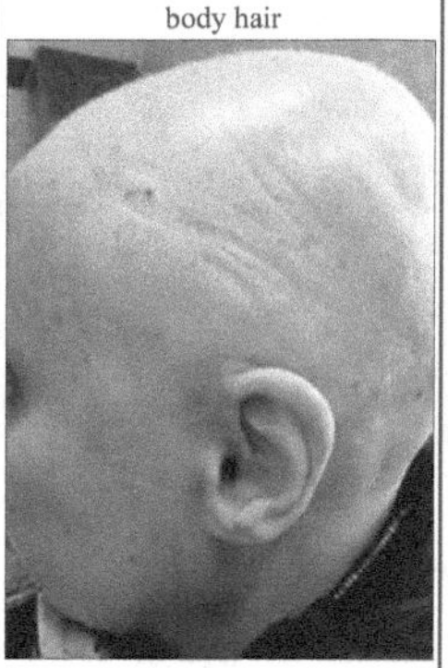	Band-like pattern over the periphery of the scalp 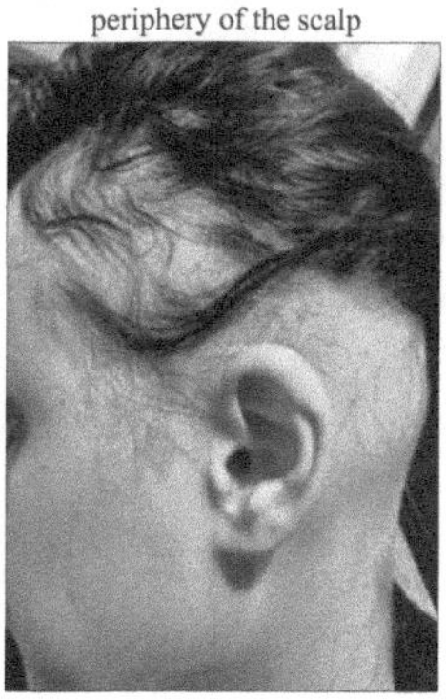

Table 2 Types of Alopecia Areata

Clinical Cases:

Case 1:

A 10-year-old girl has a history of recurrent patches of hair loss. On trichoscopic examination, findings include exclamation marks.

Exclamation Mark Hair

Stopped hair transformation leads to proximal hair constriction, which becomes lighter in color. These are considered markers of disease activity and prompt steroid use in local and systemic forms.

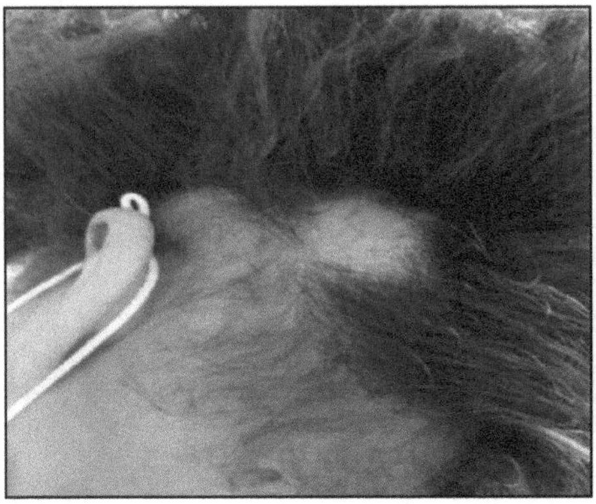

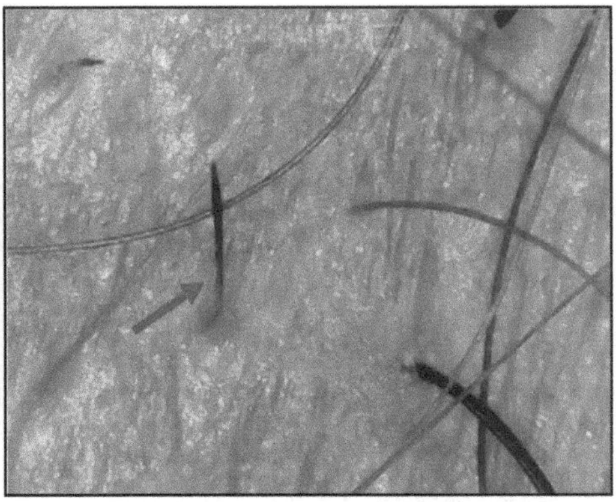

Note: Exclamation mark hairs are almost exclusive seen in Alopecia Areata

Fragile hairs that become easily broken exclusively

Case 2:

A 3-year-old girl has a history of sudden onset of diffuse patches of hair loss. Trichoscopic findings were: multiple exclamation mark hairs, black dots, and tapered hairs.

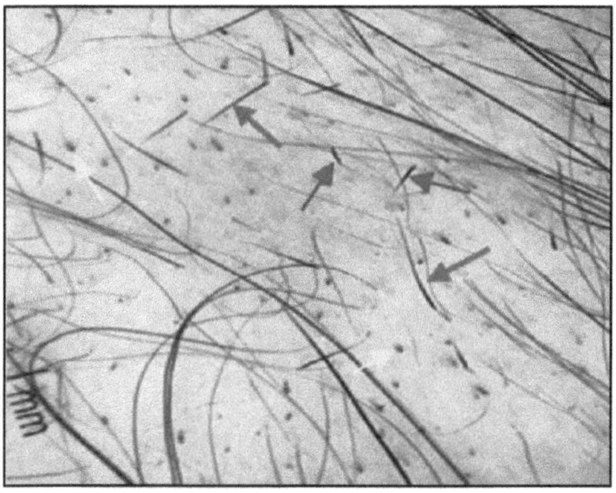

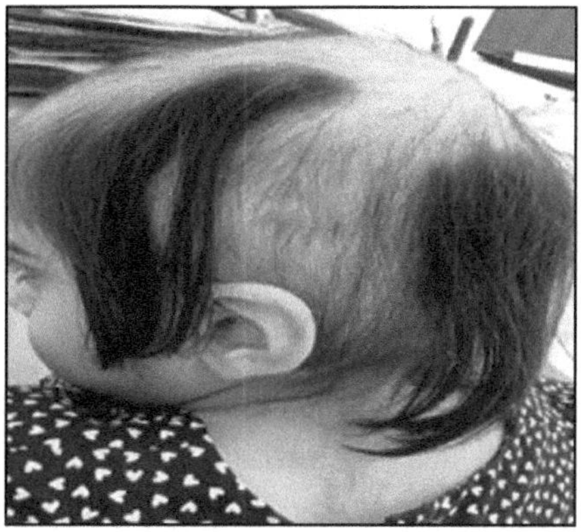

Black Dots
Macrocomedone-like round structures localized to the follicular ostium. These are residues of pigmented hairs that have broken at the level of the scalp, resembling dots on a prickly pear surface.

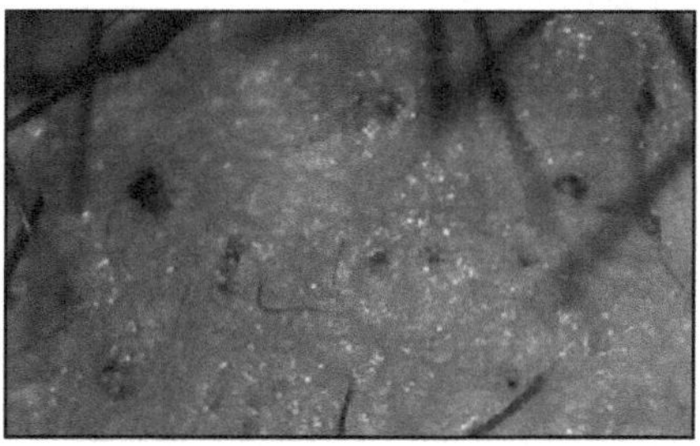

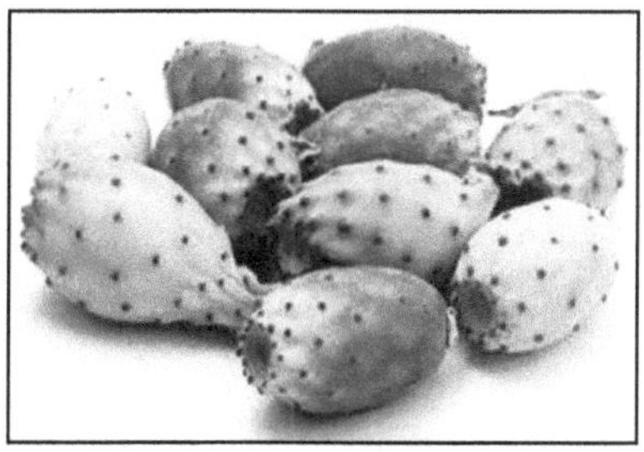

Note: Black dots are not specific for AA.

Causes of black dots:
- Inflammatory processes: Alopecia areata, dissecting cellulitis
- Hair shaft invasion: Tinea capitis
- Mechanical trauma: Trichotillomania and traction alopecia

Case 3:

A 3-year-old girl has a history of sudden onset of diffuse patches of hair loss. Trichoscopic findings were: multiple exclamation mark hairs, black dots, and tapered hairs.

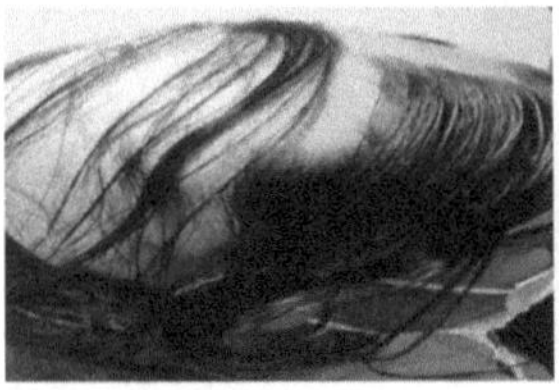
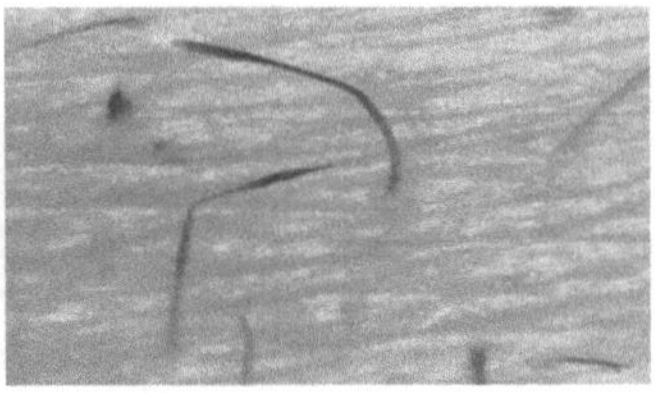
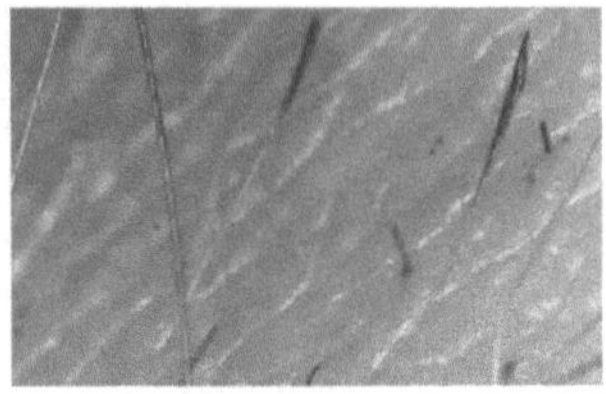

Yellow Dots

Represent distension of the affected follicular infundibulum with sebum and keratin material.

In Alopecia areata, they are rounded or polycyclic dots that vary in size and are uniform in color.

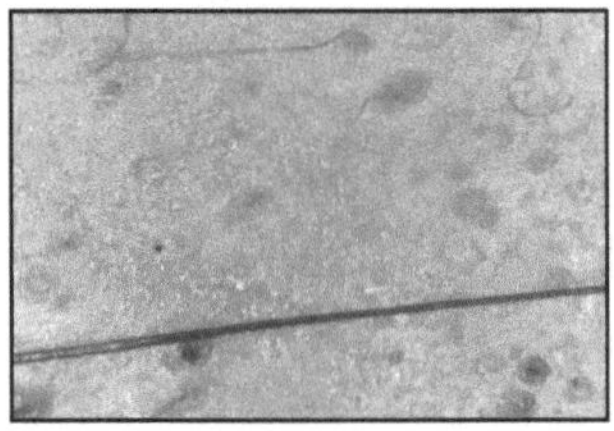

Tapered Hair (A highly specific sign for AA)

Long hair that tapers towards the root and is also lighter in color, including exclamation mark hairs and coudability hairs. These are considered markers of disease activity and are known to reflect disease exacerbation.

Tulip Hair

Short hairs with a leaf-like tulip appearance with hyperpigmentation at the distal end resulting from oblique fracture of the hair shaft distally. **It is a nonspecific feature seen in alopecia areata and trichotillomania but occurs mainly in trichotillomania.**

Case 4:

A 28-year-old female has total hair loss from the scalp and entire body.

Trichoscopic findings: multiple small and large rounded yellowish discolored dots resembling oil drops.

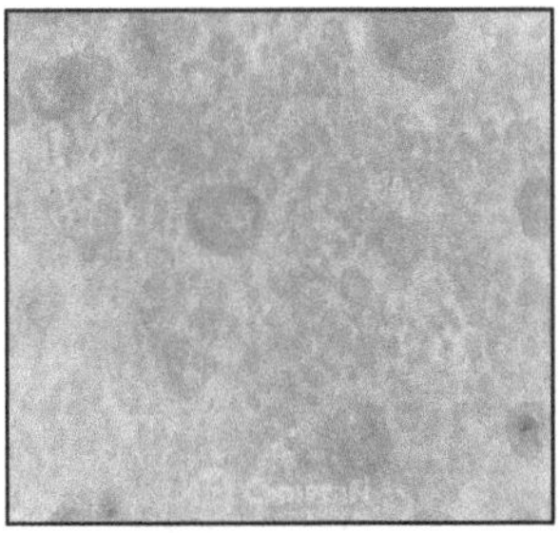
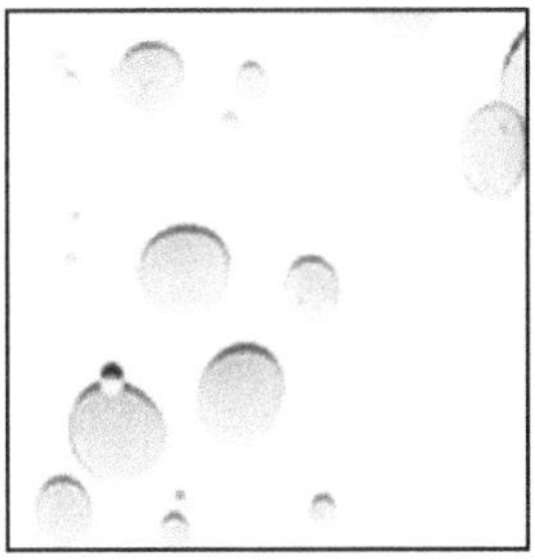
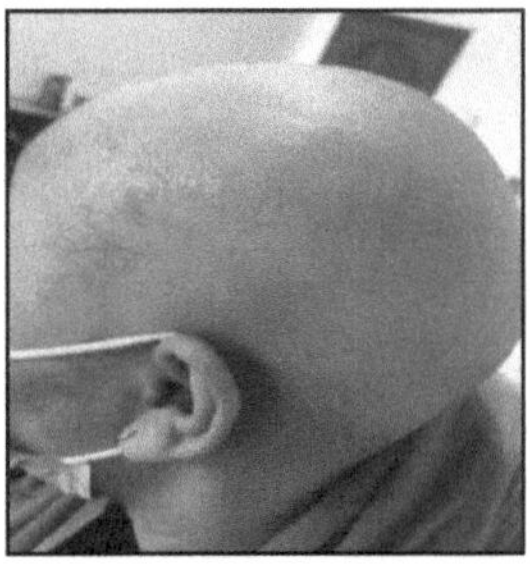

- This is a sign of severe condition
- Not specific for AA
- They are not seen in children

Case 5:

A 16-years- old female patient with ophiasis alopecia areata progress into extensive patches in 3 months duration.

Trichoscopic finding yellow dots (yellow arrow), black dots (black arrow), broken (red arrow), and comma hairs (blue arrow) indicate acute phase disease with progressive patchy AA.

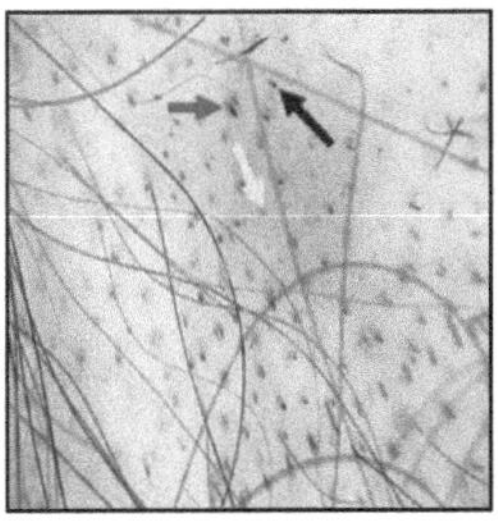
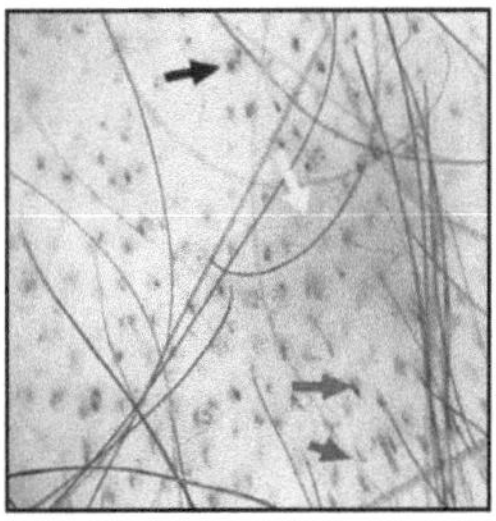
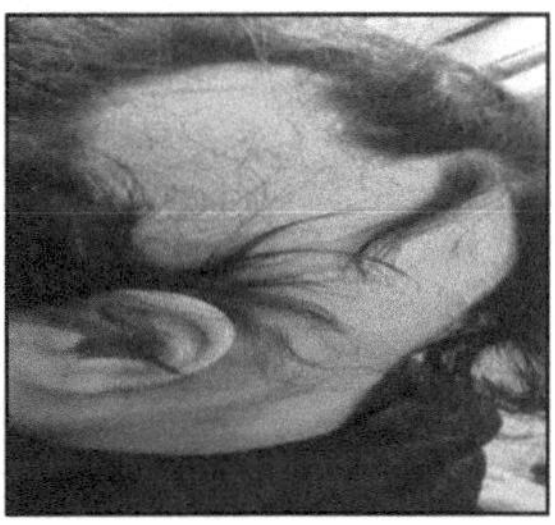

Note: Some medication staining scalp follicles causing black dots

Case 6:

A 19-years- old female patient with recurrent ophiasis alopecia areata for 5 years .

Trichoscopic findings: include yellow dots (yellow arrow) and exclamation mark hairs (red arrow).

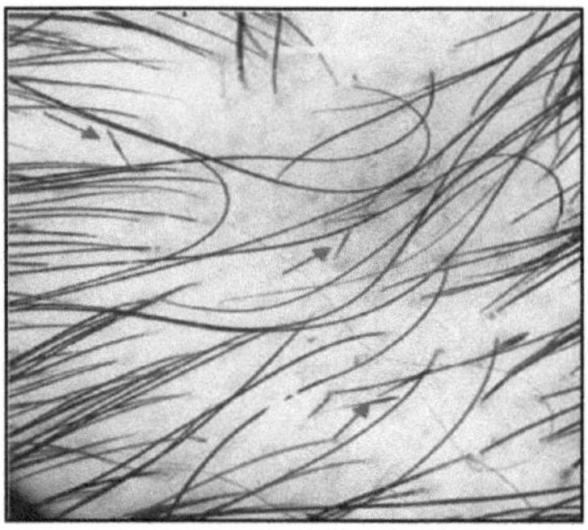

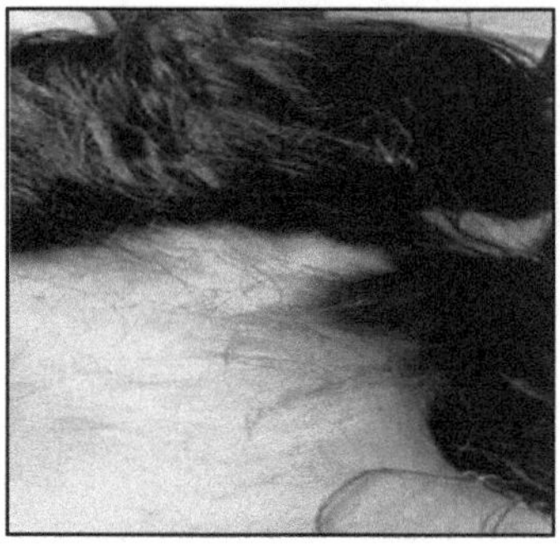

Case 7:

Diabetic young male patient has single patch of AA for 2 months .

Trichoscopic findings: Tulip hair (green arrows), exclamation mark hairs (red arrow) and, broken hairs (blue arrow) .

Tulip hairs occur with exclamation hairs; this feature is seen in alopecia areata.

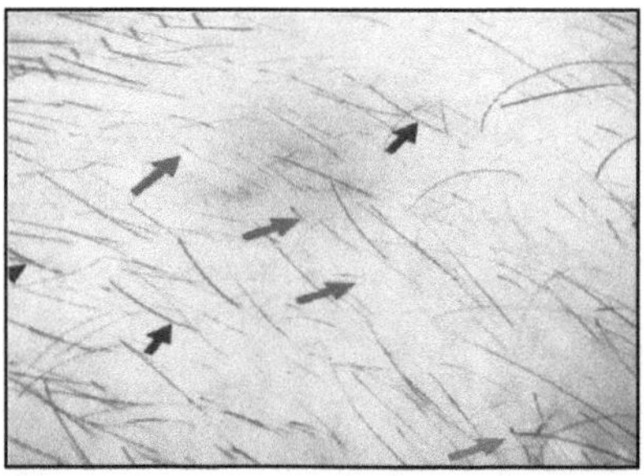

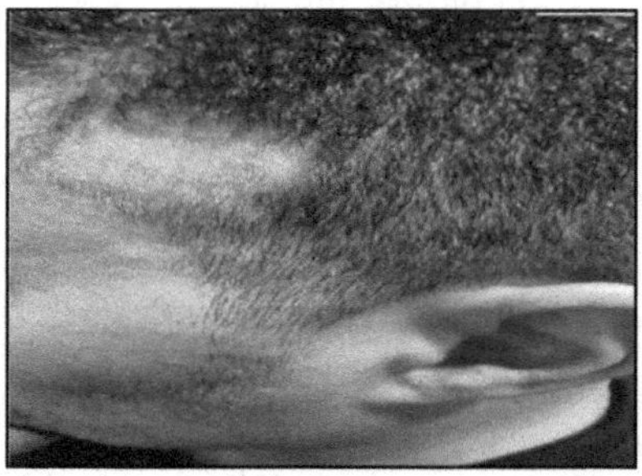

Short broken hairs can be seen in:

- Alopecia areata: in AA are dystrophic hair produced by the least severely affected follicles
- Tinea capitus
- Trichotillomania

Case 8:

A 19-years- old female patient presents with recurrent multiple patches of AA.

Trichoscopic findings: broken hairs at the similar level (white arrow), exclamation mark hairs (red arrow).

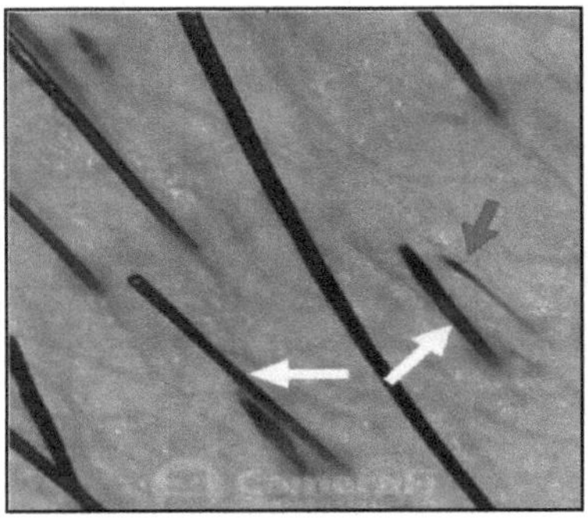

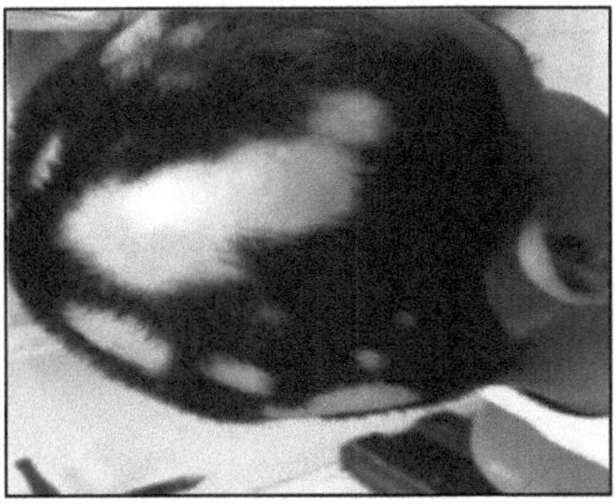

Case 9:

An 8-year-boy diagnosed as case of alopecia universalis for 5 years associated with nail pitting .

Trichoscopic findings: Black dots, white dots, elbow sign.

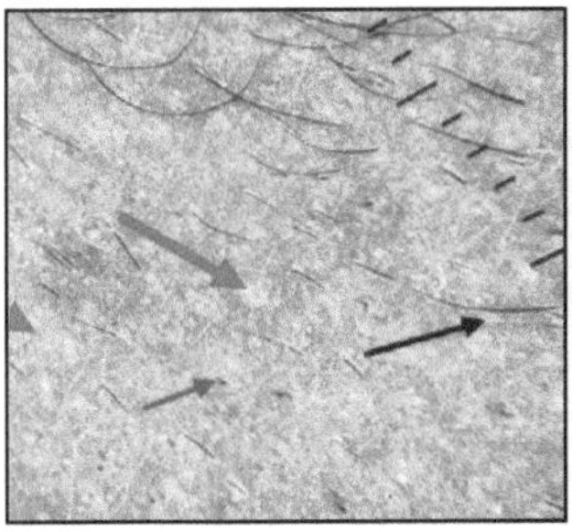

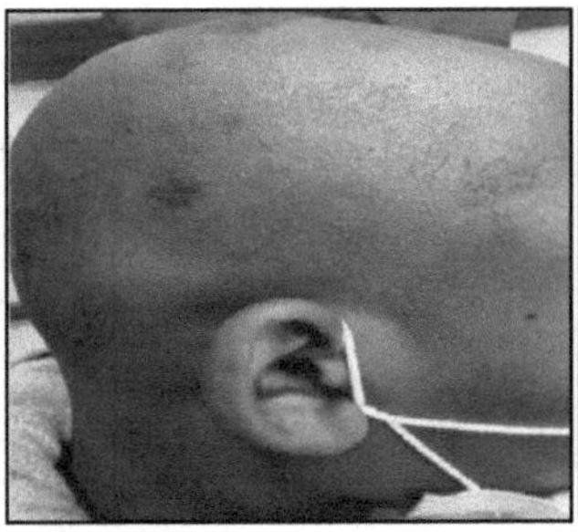

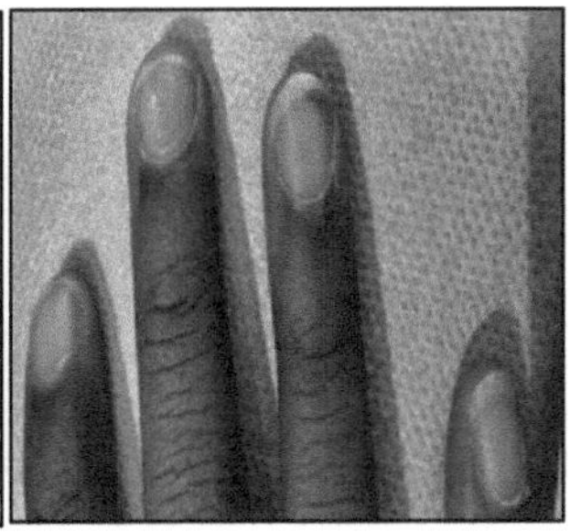

Note:

white dots:

• Small irregular areas of fibrosis • Small regular it is seen in dark skin, corresponds to follicular and sweat glands openings

Case 10:

An 8-year-boy diagnosed as case of alopecia universalis for 5 years associated with nail pitting .

Trichoscopic findings: Black dots, white dots, elbow sign.

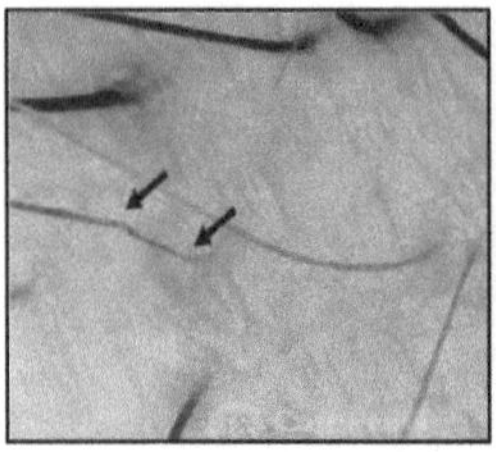
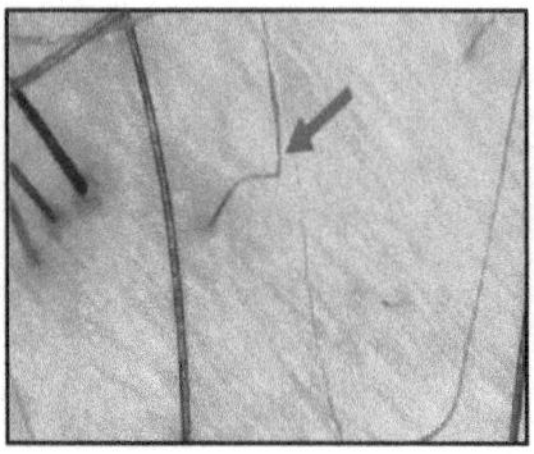
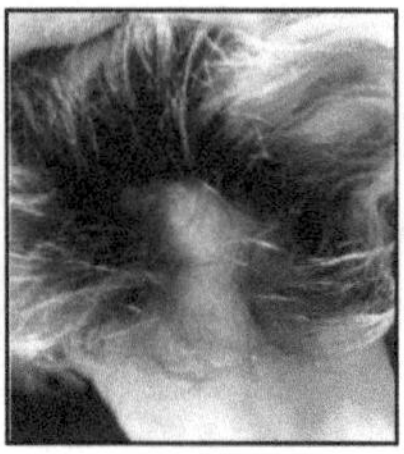
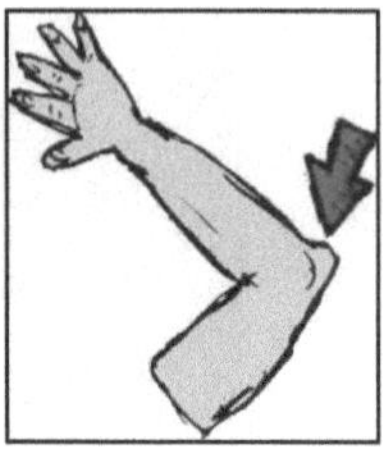

Elbow hair

Coudability hair (or elbow hair) is bent hair with a narrowed proximal end. It appears in follicles affected by early inflammation in alopecia areata because of hair shaft thinning.

Pohl-Pinkus.

Monilethrix-like hair is characterized by constrictions on the hair shaft placed at irregular intervals, which are vulnerable to hair breakage, commonly seen in AA but less in cicatricial alopecia, and localized hereditary hypotrichosis, as well as chemotherapy.

A tapered hair corresponds to a very long Pohl-Pinkus's constriction. Technically, hairs that are thin at the proximal end and become normal distally are called tapered hair.

Pohl-Pinkus's constriction (monilethrix-like hair)

- Alopecia areata
- Chemotherapy
- Cicatricial alopecia
- Severe blood loss
- Malnutrition
- Localized hereditary hypotrichosis

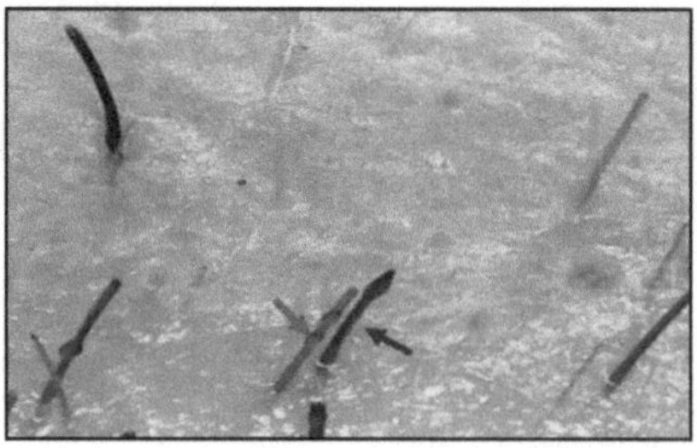

Note:

Always search for exclamation mark hairs and elbow sign at the margin of AA patch

Case 11:

A 62-year-old diabetic man has sudden onset of bitemporal patchy alopecia .

Trichoscopic findings: black dots (red arrow), black arrow shows preservation of the honey-comb-like pigment network, exclamation mark hairs (green arrow).

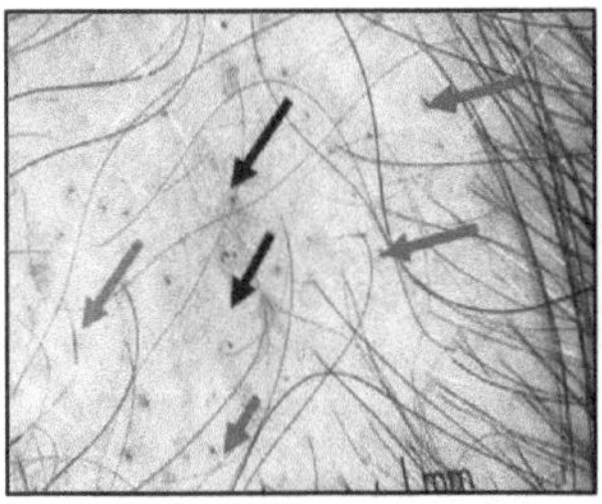

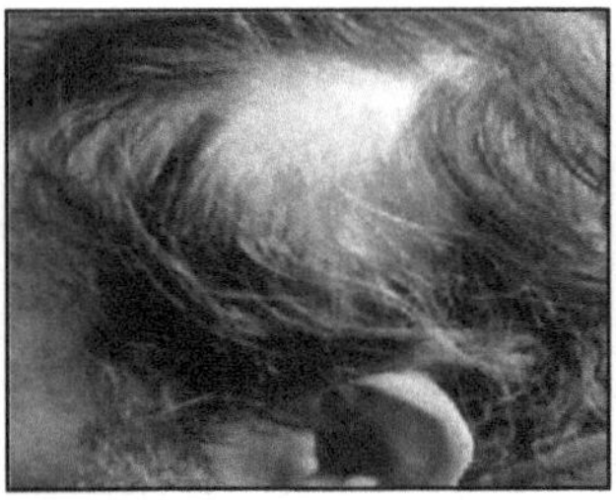

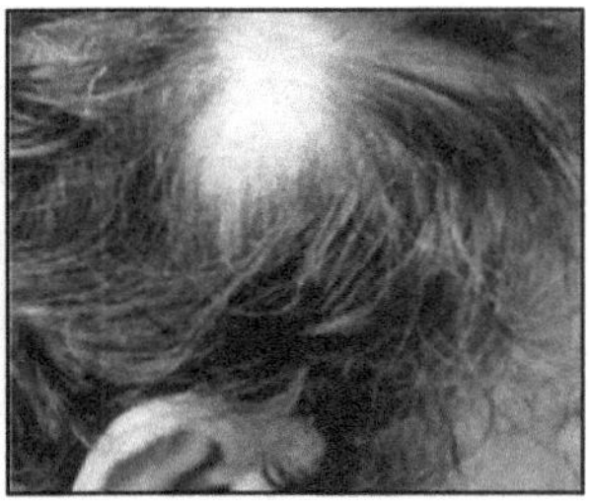

Reticulate hyperpigmentation

- It is a relatively uncommon dermatological pattern.
- It is used to describe brown-colored areas that manifest in a lacy or network-like distribution, corresponding to the rete ridge pattern of the epidermis.

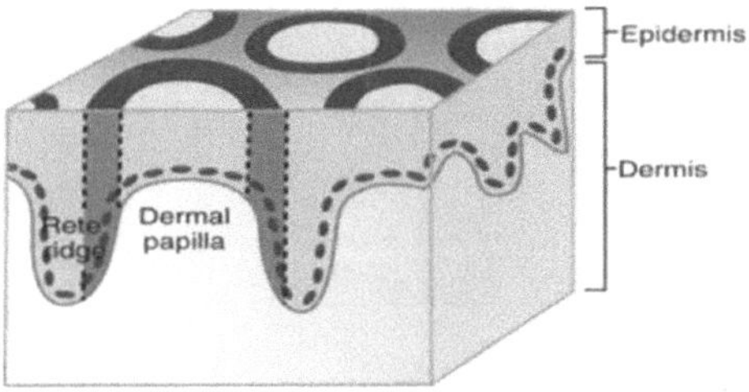

Case 12:

A 10-year-male presented with recurrent patchy& ophiasis alopecia

Trichoscopic features: split hair (yellow arrow), perifollicular scales (green arrow), tapered hairs (black arrow), micro-exclamation mark shorter than 1-2mm (red arrow), black dots.

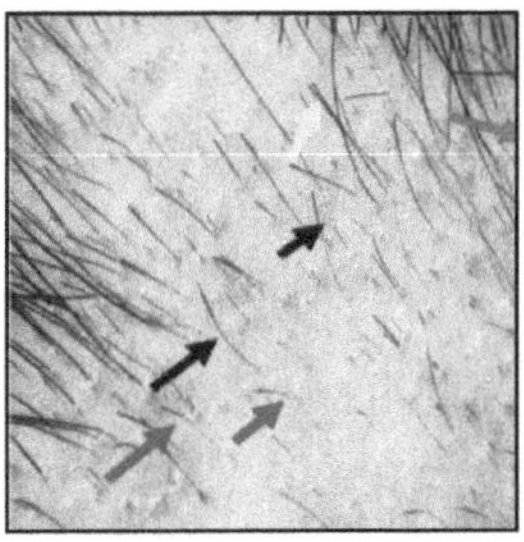

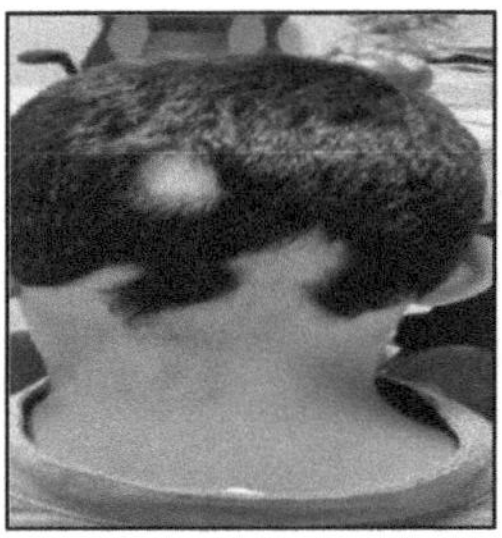

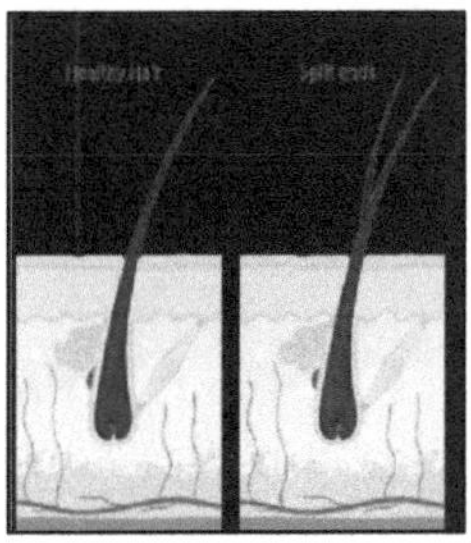

Trichoptilosis (split hair ends)
It is used to describe distal splitting and damage of the hair shaft; it may be seen in patients with AA and in individuals using cosmetic-damaging agents such as straighteners.

Case 13:

A 15-year-female has extended patches of hair loss on vertex which responded and hair growth after using local dithranol cream 0.4% .

Trichoscopic features: during treatment respond, pig-tail hair (black arrow) and up right regrowing hair (red arrow).

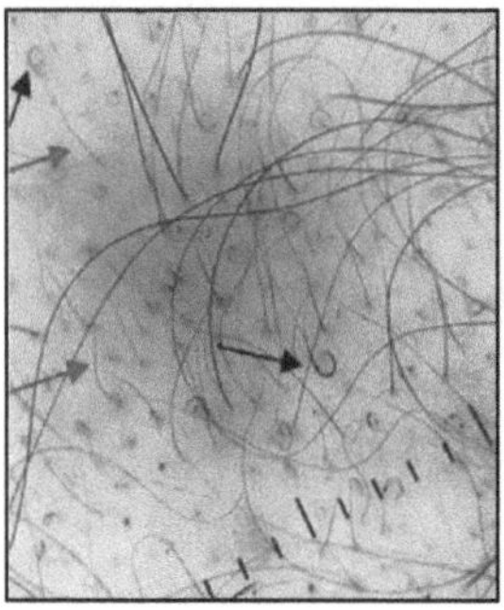

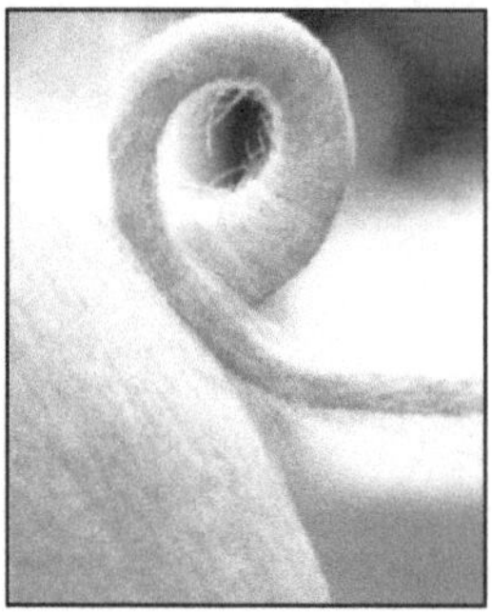

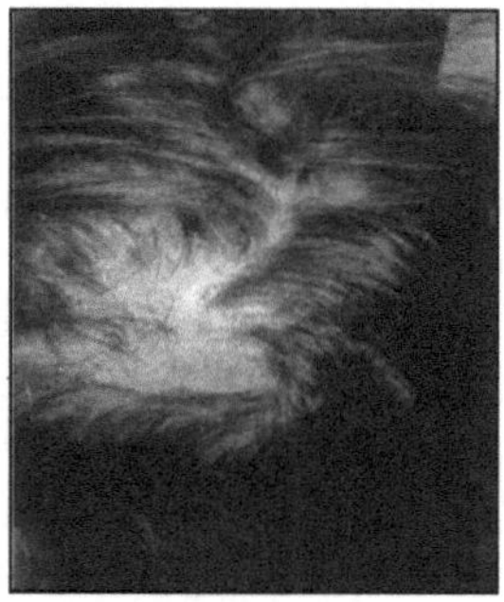

Pigtail hairs:
Short, twisted hair representing regrowing hair looks like a tail.

Upright re-growing hair	**Vellus hair**
Short3-5mm	Very short, <3mm
Thin > 50μm	Very thin, <30 μm
Normally pigmented	Hypopigmented
upright position	Way shape
Firm appearance	Weak appearance
Pointed distal end	Blurred distal ends

Case14:

A 6-year- old boy presented with recurrent alopecia at the scalp margins and multiple patchy alopecia.

Trichoscopic findings: Exclamation mark; yellow arrow, broken hairs; red arrow, scalp erythema, red dots; blue arrow.

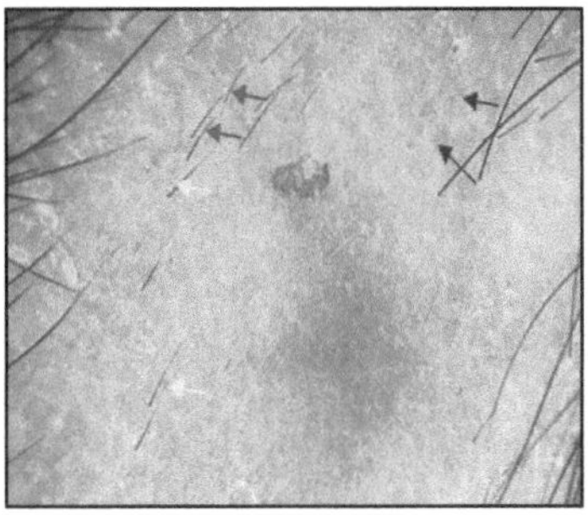

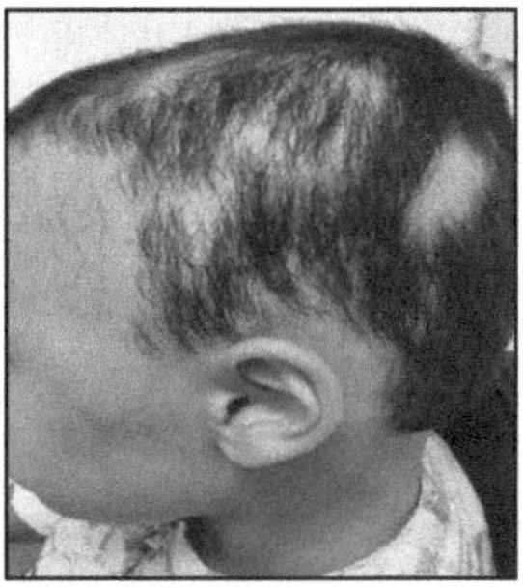

Trichoscopic Findings of Alopecia by Disease Stage

Stage	**Findings**
Active Stage	Broken hair, Coudability sign, Exclamation mark, Black dots
Stable Stage	Yellow dots, Short vellus hair, Circle hair (short vellus hair which tends to become coiled hair)
Regrowth Stage	Upright regrowing hair, Pigtail hair
Others	Pseudomonilethrix (irregular and multiple constrictions of the hair shaft)

1.2 Acute Diffuse and Total Alopecia (ADTA) and Alopecia Areata Incognita (AAI)

A synonym for self-regressing severe alopecia areata.

- Lacks the typical patchy hair loss seen in classical alopecia areata and presents with an acute onset of diffuse hair loss
- Shows rapid hair transition from anagen to telogen
- It is commonly reported in young females
- It has a duration from 2 to 20 weeks
- Has a rapid progression with a short recovery time and a favorable prognosis
- It is confirmed only by histopathology, as trichoscopic features are not specific

Numerous yellow dots are the most frequent pattern, either empty yellow dots or yellow dots with vellus hairs. Small hair regrowth with the presence of pigtail hair is exclusive to AAI.

Case- 15:

A15-year- old female who presented with sudden onset of diffuse hair loss within one week. Trichoscopic findings: yellow dots; green arrow, vellus hair; blue arrow, pig tail hair; white arrow, up right regrowing hair; red arrow, dark line; black arrow .

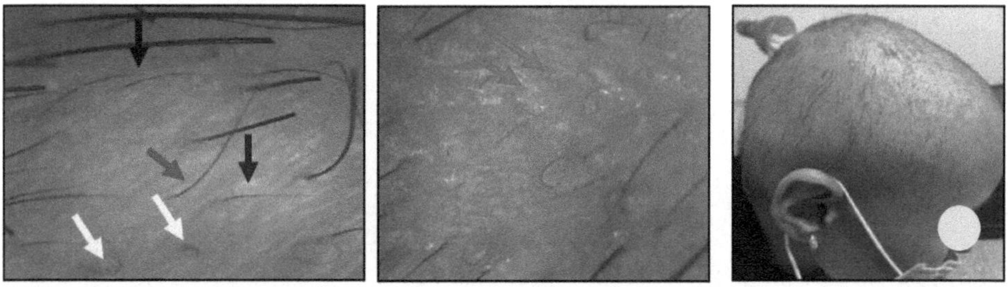

Note:

Short vellus hairs, which are thin and non-pigmented correlates with regrowth phase, dark lines are present commonly in AAI.

Case- 16:

A57-year- female presented with diffuse hair loss for one year, she had history of patchy hair loss 20 years ago :

- Picture of ADTA like telogen effluvium, androgenetic alopecia.
- Trichoscopic findings: multiple grouped yellow dots; black arrows.

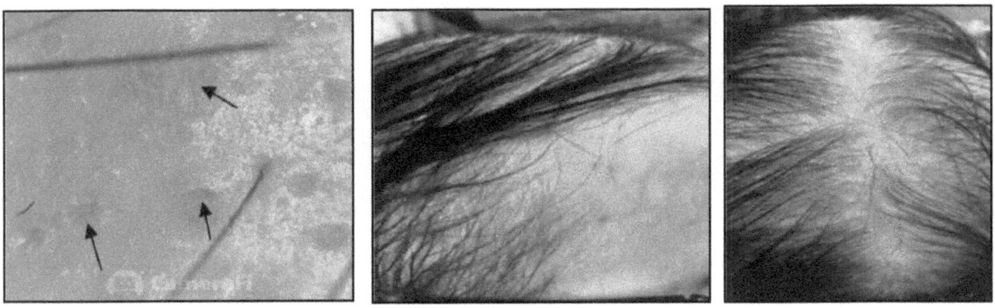

1.3 Diffuse hair loss

1.3.1 Telogen Effluvium (TE):

- Anagen hairs are actively growing hair, while telogen hairs are resting hair. If there is some kind of stress to the body, it can cause up to 70% of anagen hairs to precipitate into the telogen phase, thus causing hair loss.
- On trichoscopy, TE is a diagnosis of exclusion based mainly on typical clinical history and examination.
- T E Characterized by decreased hair density, minimal or no variation of hair shaft diameter, even in the chronic forms, short regrowing hair, also called upright regrowing hair, and a single hair shaft emerging from a follicular unit.
- Peripilar halo: peripilar brown discoloration around the hair follicle, which is due to perifollicular inflammation.
- Focal Atrichia.

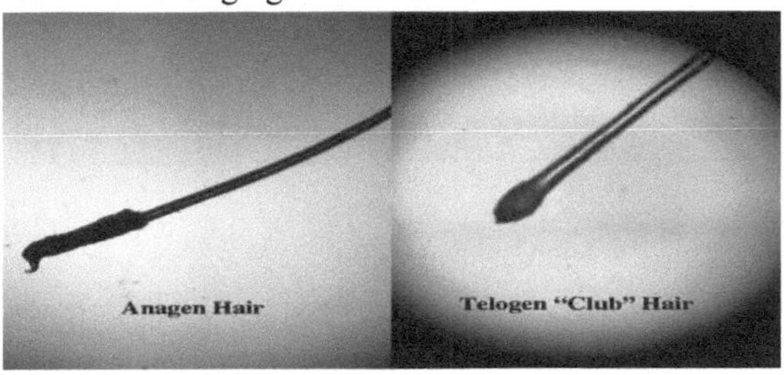

Case- 17:

28 years old postpartum lactating mother presented with sudden onset of hair shedding. Up right re growing (white arrow) and no variation of hair shafts diameter hair (yellow arrow).

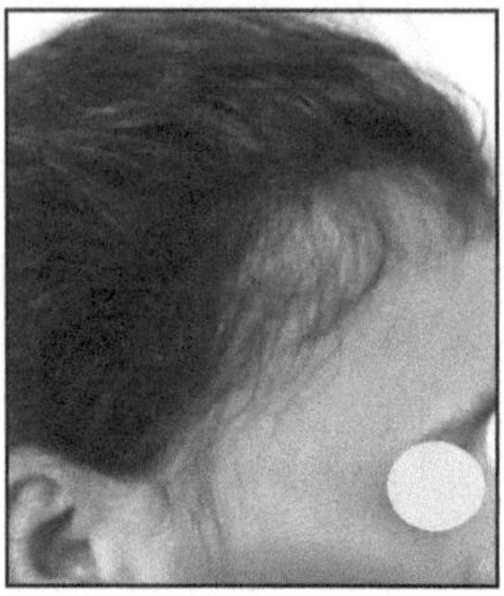

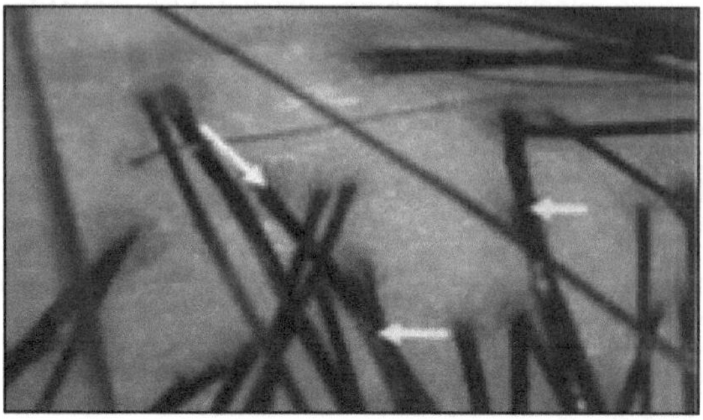

Case- 18:

A 32-year- old female who presented with sudden onset of diffuse hair loss after crash diet with low laboratory parameters for ferritin and vitamin D levels.

Trichoscopic findings: Peri pilar halo; green arrow, up right regrowing hair (thin tip and grow thicker at base); yellow arrow.

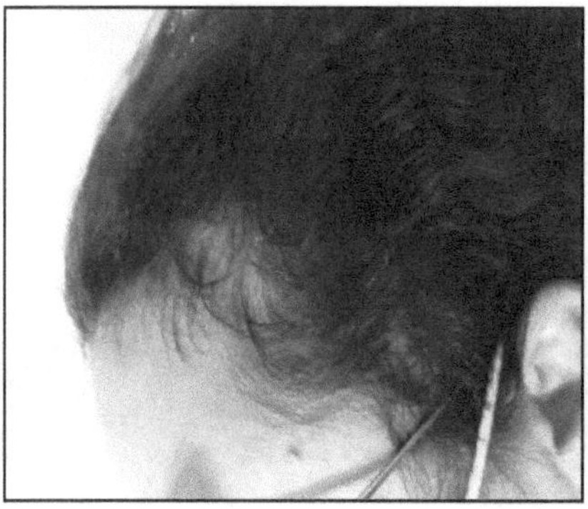

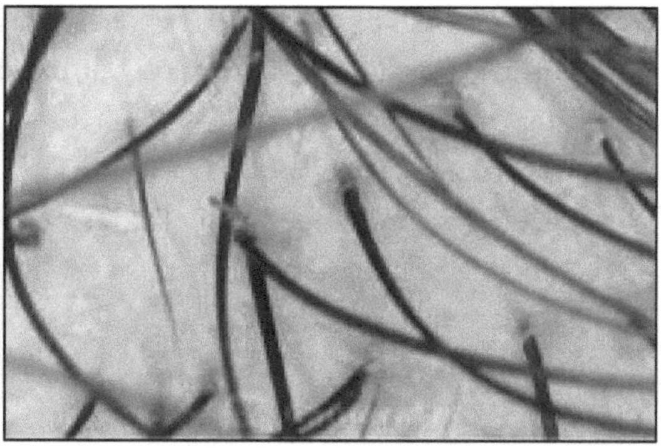

1.3.2 Anagen Effluvium:

Usually seen after exposure to chemotherapy or radiotherapy

- Trichoscopic features: black dots, yellow dots, tapering hair, Pohl-Pinkus's constriction, monilethrix–like hair, circular hair, peripilar sign, which is related to perifollicular infiltration.
- Tulip-like hair proximally is normal in color and thickness due to distal hair fall during chemotherapy induction; the shaft progressively narrows, which ends as a dark tip.
- Flame hair.

Case- 19:

Anagen effliuvum in 56year old female, she received 3 cycles of chemotherapy for breast cancer .

On trichoscopy :

Tulipoid hair: proximal portion of the hair shaft (red arrow) indicates the cessation of chemotherapy and restart follicular activity. Distal portion of the hair shaft (yellow arrow) marks the onset of chemotherapy causing constriction and tapering, resulting in the distal tip falling off to form tulip-like tip.

Elbow hair (white arrow), black dots (green arrow), red dots (blue arrows), peripilar sign (black arrows), Tulipoid hair (yellow arrow).

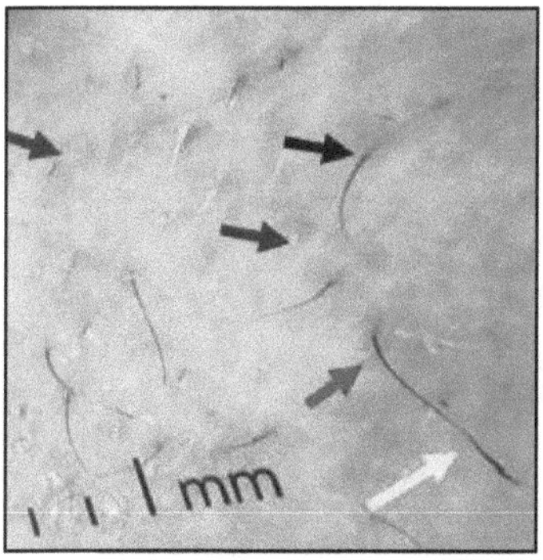

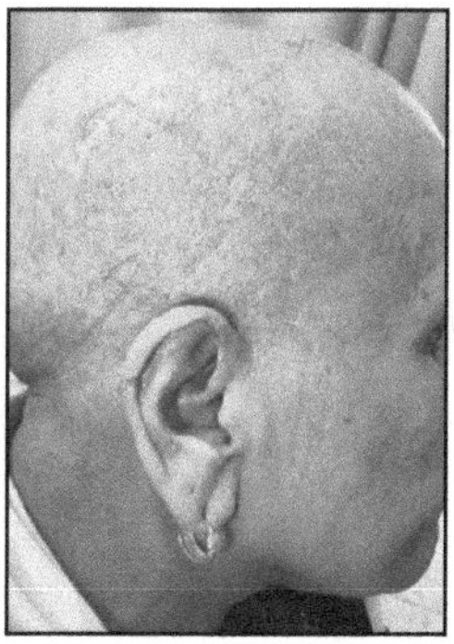
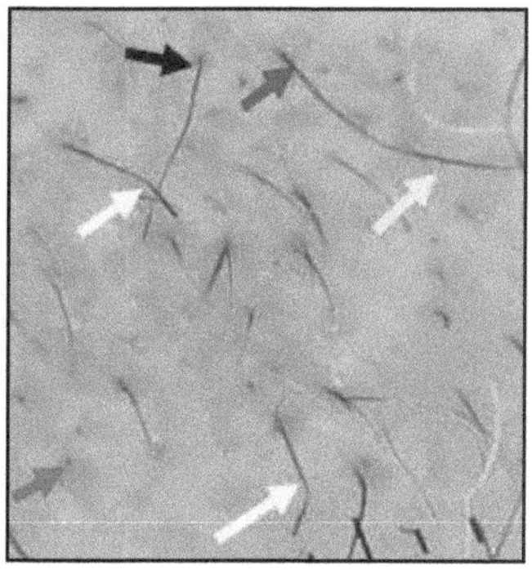

1.3.3 Androgenetic Alopecia:

It has differences in distribution between male and female, but trichoscopic features are the same, which occur mainly in the frontal region, including:

- Decrease hair density.
- Increase variation in hair diameter by more than 20% looks like trees in the forest
- Empty hair follicle.
- Yellow dots are four in number on four trichoscopic fields.
- Variation in the number of hairs in each follicular unit.
- Brown perifollicular halo, which is mostly noted in the vertex region and is very specific.
- More than six thin re-growing hairs in the frontal scalp.
- Focal atrichia: it means atrophic follicles, correlated to the advanced stage.
- Honeycomb pigmented network in sun–exposed scalp, seen in severe cases.
- Pinpoint white dots in sun-exposed tanned scalp.

Case- 20:

A 28-years- old female patient presents with 4 years gradual diffuse hair thinning and decreased density.

Trichoscopic findings: yellow dots with thin vellus hair (yellow arrow), single hair piercing hair follicle (red arrows), hair shaft diversity, peripilar sign; 1mm in diameter around the emergence of the hair shaft (blue arrows).

Thinned hair shafts: anisotrichosis and yellow dots indicate sever miniaturization.

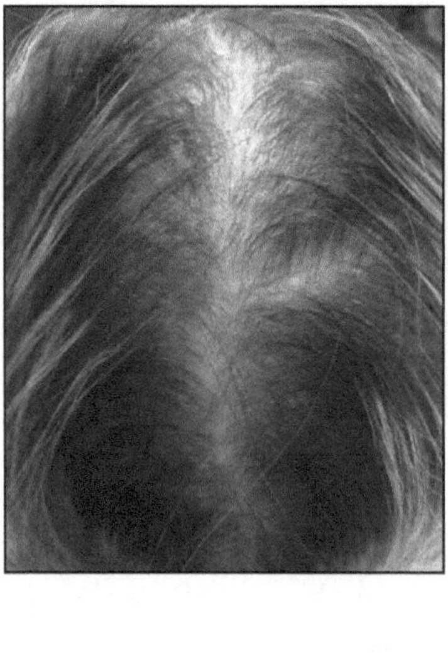

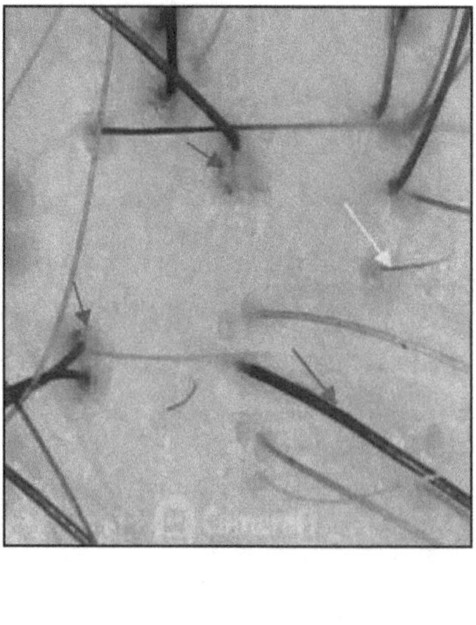

Case- 21

A 40-years- old famale patient presents a gradual diffuse hair thining and decreased hair density with wide central parting.
Trichoscopic findings: vellus hair (blue arrow), yellow dots (white arrow), single hair piercing hair follicle (red arrow).

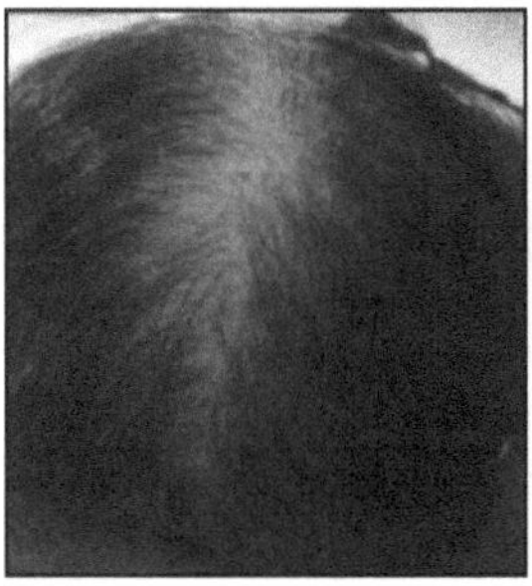
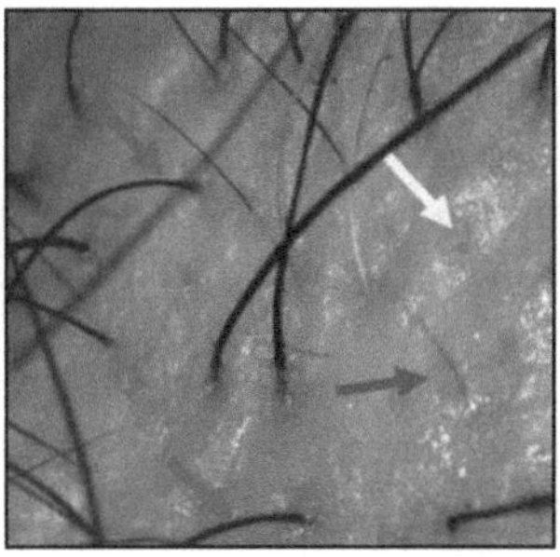
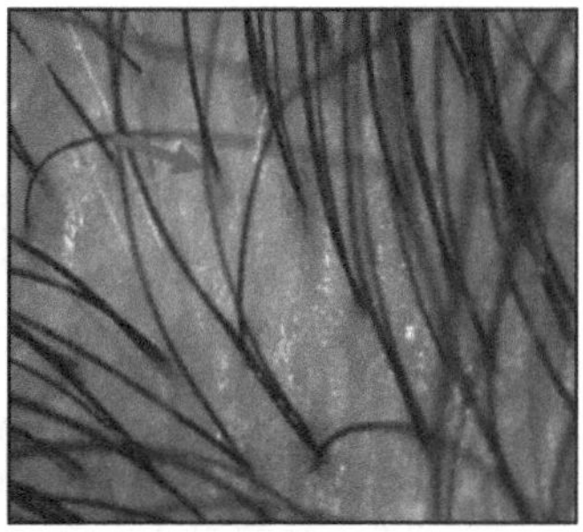

Note:

- Advice patient avoid hair washing at least 2 days before AGA examination
- Avoid black dye hair staining as it may confused with black dots

Feature	Telogen effluvium-TE	Androgenetic alopecia-AGA
Anisiotrichosis	Not present	Present
Vellus-like hair	Not present	Present
Single hair containing a follicular unit in the frontal area	Present	Common
Upright regrowing hair	Common	Not present
Empty hair follicle (including yellow dots)	Present	Present
Peripilar sign	Present	Common
Predominance of abnormalities in the frontal region	Not present	Common

1.3.4 Trichotellomania:

The presenting sign is single or multiple ill-defined patches of incomplete alopecia with underlying compulsive psychological disturbance.
The vertex and parietal regions are the most common sites where all characteristic features are seen under the dermoscope due to the repeated traumatic fractures of the hair shafts.

Trichoscopic diagnosis of trichotellomania is difficult because there are no diagnostic criteria.

- **Broken hairs** are short hairs with irregular and ragged distal ends that are most often caused by mechanical force
- **Black dots** and black dots in yellow dots, by which you can differentiate from AA
- **Exclamation mark hairs** in patients with AA have frayed distal ends, whereas most exclamation mark hairs in trichotillomania patients have blunt distal ends and dark proximal ends.
- **V shape** sign when two hairs emerge from a single hair unit are broken at the same level (Ballerina hairs). It may be seen in all regrowing hair after shaving.

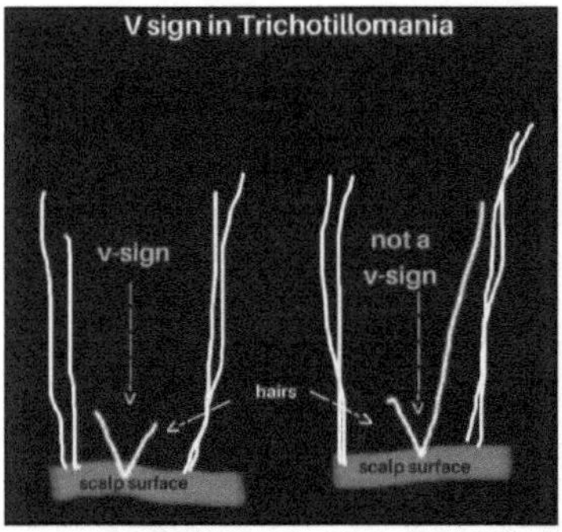

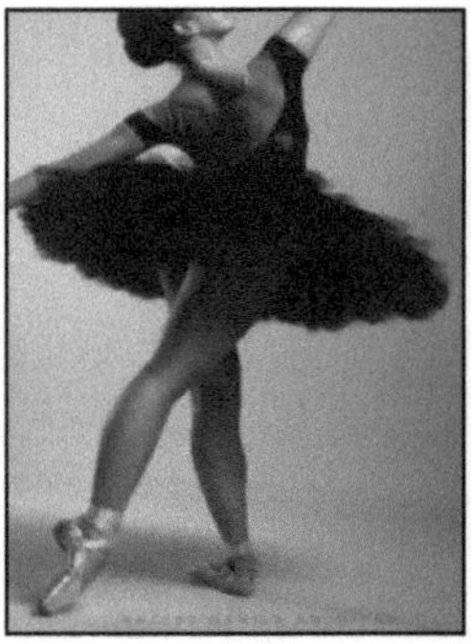
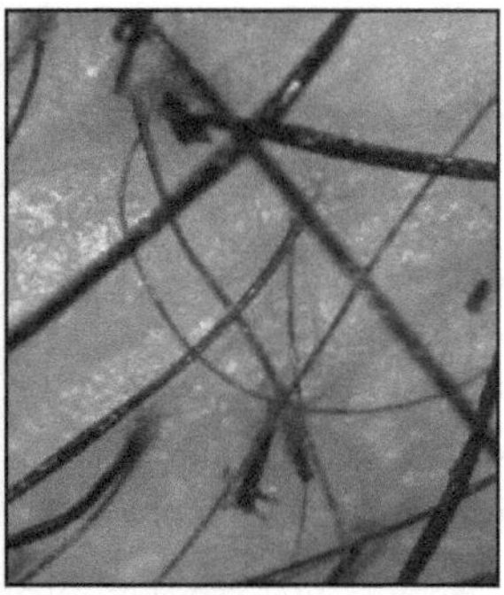

- **Hair powder**: destroyed hair residues because of repeated pulling.
- **Mac sign**: distal hair end appears rough and dilated while proximal hair is pigmented. Have seen in some patients that, due to strong pulling hairs, it is regarded as a good sign to differentiate it from alopecia areata (exclamation mark).
- **Flame figure:** due to severe mechanical pulling of hair, it appears dark and bulbous proximally.
- **Hook hair:** appears as a coiled shape with a blunt end due to elasticity recoil when applying strong tension on hair, differentiated from pigtail hair, which is circular, and regrowing hair.

- **i hair sign**: a short hair with an accentuated distal end, resembling the letter i. This sign is considered a positive prognostic marker in patients with AA and trichotillomania.
- **Trichoptilosis:** longitudinal split hair at ends; it is not pathognomic for any alopecia type.
- **Tulip hair:** proximally, it is light in color, while distally, it appears dark due to an oblique fracture of the distal hair shaft, which is a nonspecific feature also seen in AA.

Case- 22

A 23-years- old female has recurrent hair pulling and plucking result. Findings on trichoscopy: Microhaemorrhages around the infundibulum and perifollicular areas (yellow arrows), i hair sign (red arrow), and yellow dots (blue arrow).

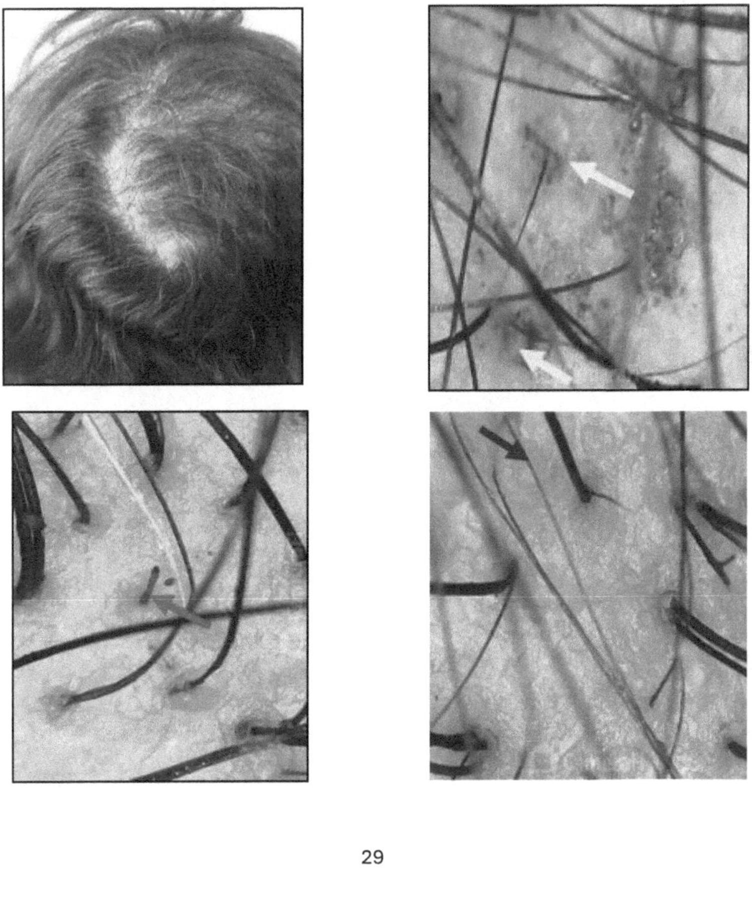

Case- 23

An 8-years- old girl has irregular patches of alopecia with broken hair on eye brows for 2-months

Trichoscopic findings shows: Broken hair at different level (red arrows), flame figure synonymous burnt matchstick sign: wavy cone shaped hair residue (black arrow), i- hair (yellow arrows), Mac sign (blue arrow) and Trichoptilosis (white arrow).

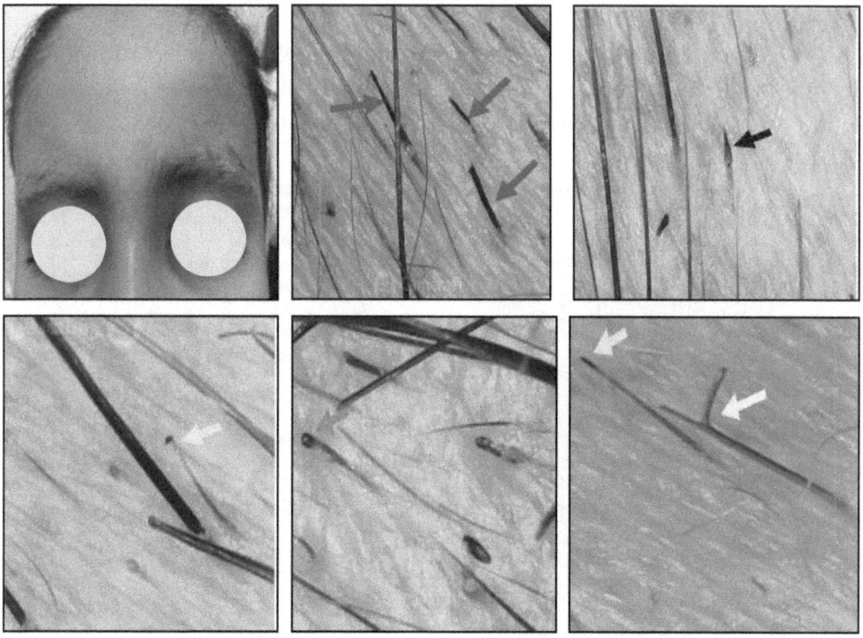

Case- 24

An 11-years- old girl has large patch of hair loss on vertex and bitemporal regions for 6-months.

Trichoscopic findings:
Black dots red arrow, flam figure (yellow arrow), hook hair (black arrow), trichopetilosis (blue arrow), v shape (white arrow), hook hair (green arrow), and Exclamation mark (purple arrow).

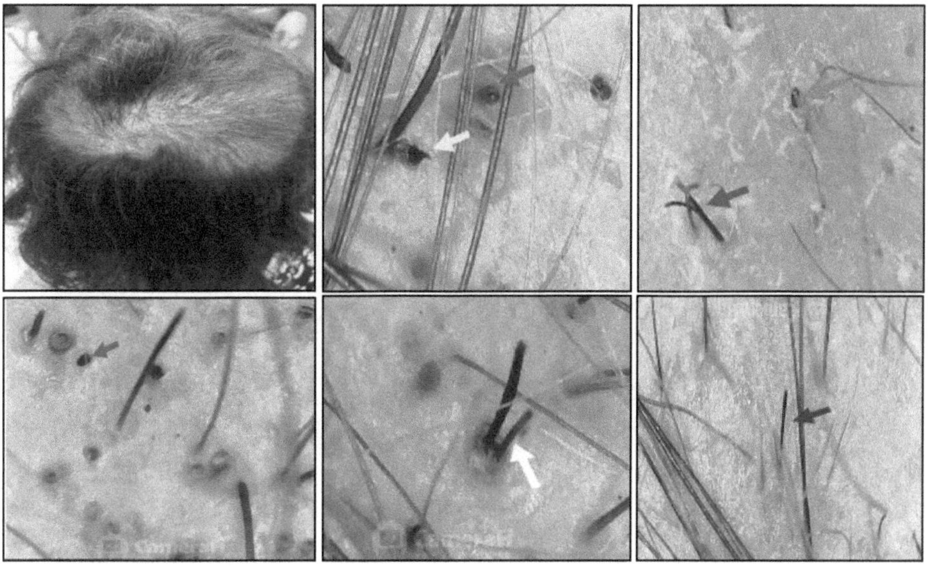

Note:
coiled hair equal to hook hair because has hook -like occurs after fracturing, the remaining part of the hair coils irregularly

Case- 25

A 16-years- old girl has patch of hair loss and decreased density involving the entire scalp.
Trichoscopic findings: Flamme figure (red arrows), v shape (blue arrow).

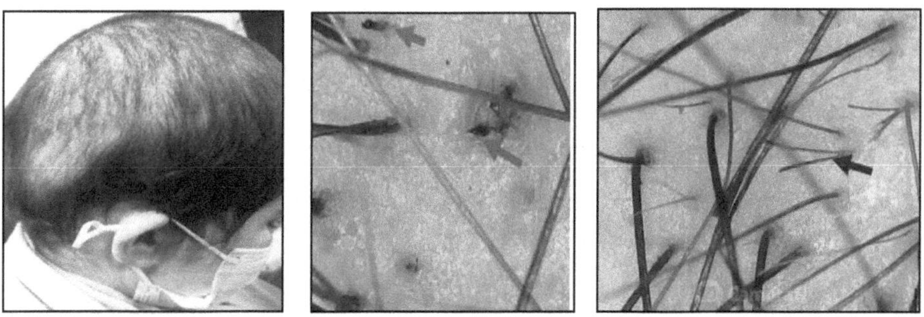

Case- 26

A 12-years- old girl has patch of hair loss involving the crown and occipital scalp
Trichoscopic findings: Hook hair (red arrows), v shape (blue arrow).

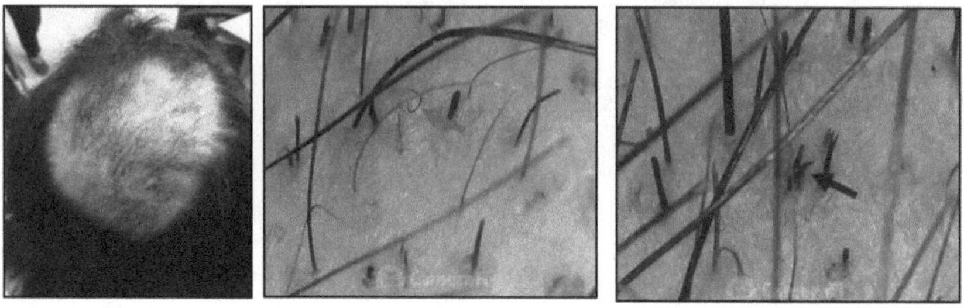

Case- 27

An 18-years- old girl has patch of hair loss on frontal rgion of the scalp for 2 months Trichoscopic findings: V shape (red arrow), microheamorrahge (blue arrow).

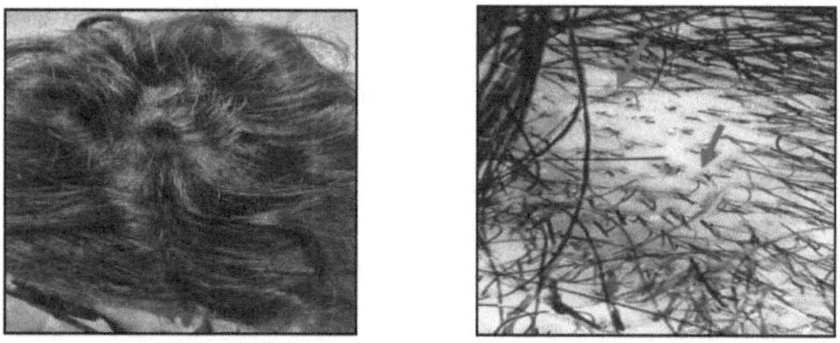

Case- 28

An 18-years- old girl has patch of hair loss on frontal rgion of the scalp for 2 months.

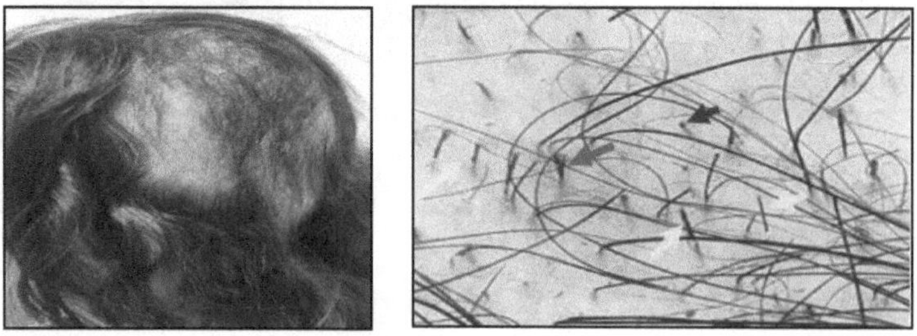

Trichoscopic features common to AA& trichotelomania
• **Micro-exclamation mark** • **Black dots** • **trichoptillosis**

Traction alopecia-TA

TA is defined as hair loss caused by repetitive or continuous and prolonged tension applied to the margin of the scalp, either due to occupational behavioral patterns, such as ballerinas or traditional hair styling, that induce hair loss and later produce scarring alopecia.

Trichoscopic features:

- Reduce hair density
- Vellus hairs
- Broken hairs
- Short regrowing hairs
- Fringe sign: vellus hairs retained at the edge of the affected area in the marginal-type tractional alopecia
- Yellow dots
- Perifollicular brown pigmentation
- Hair cast
- Irregular small white dots
- Extravasated blood

Case- 29

A 6-years- old black skinned girl presents has progressive hair line thining of the frontal abd temporal region with witish scales which may miss diagnosed as nits. Trichoscopic findings: Perifollicular scales (black arrow). black dot (red arrow), vellus hair (blue arrow), perifollicual brown discoloration (purple arrow), and peipilar cast (black arrow).

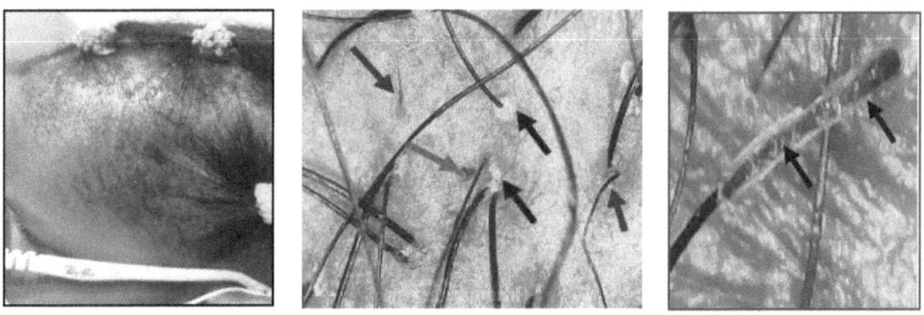

Note:

- **Hair casts** (pseudonits): are 2-7 mm longe, freely movable, gray-white cylindrical wrapped around the proximal hair shaft at the periphery of the lesion
- **Peripilar cast** represent to the detached hyperkeratotic and parakeratotic cells inner root sheath
- Hair cast may be a secondary phenomenon during psoriasis, seborrheic dermatitis or lichen plano pilaris
- Idiopathic hair cast may be observed in healthy individuals

Case- 30

A 7-years- old girl presents with gradual decreased frontal hair density

Trichoscopic findings: perifollicular scales (red arrow), yellow dots (black arrows), trichonodosis (white arrow), white dots (blue arrow).

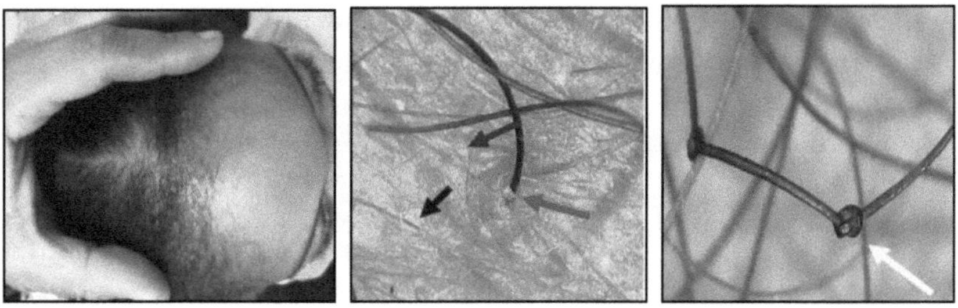

2. Scarring Alopecia

Lichen Planopilaris:

- The most common cause of scarring alopecia.
- A slow-onset and gradual progression condition is typically seen in adults and is very rare in children.
- Clinically, patients present with multiple patches of scarring alopecia.

Trichoscopic features:

Active lesions:

- Perifollicular white prominent scales are arranged in a tubular-like structure.
- Perifollicular dark brown violaceous pigmentation.

- Hair cast.
- Perifollicular erythema.
- Elongated linear blood vessels.

Inactive lesions:

- Irregular large white dots.
- White patches indicate fibrosis.
- Milky red areas (strawberry ice cream color) due to the new onset of fibrosis.
- Decreased hair density and absence of follicular openings.
- Tufted hair, two to four hairs surrounded by scales.
- Pili torti.

Case- 31

A 63-years- old female hypothyroid patient presents with large patch of hair loss on vertex was preceded by trauma 11 years ago .

Trichoscopic findings :

Perifollicular white scales surrounded by violet, brown halo (green arrows), hair cast (yellow arrow), blue gray dots (red arrows), white dots (blue arrow) tend to merge and become confluent, and they form ivory white areas (black arrow).

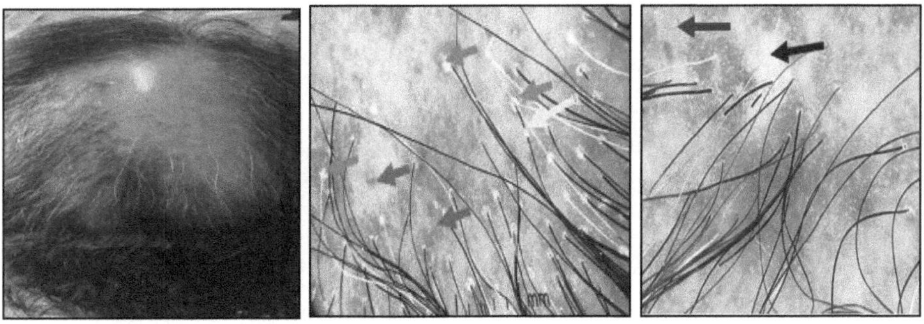

- Violet- brown areas are common in inflammatory lesions, correspond to the pigment incontinence seen on histopathology
- Ivory white areas (red arrow) indicate follicular openings fibrosis.

Case- 32

A 33-years- old female hypothyroid patient presents multiple patches of hair loss on the scalp for 3 years associated with hyperpigmented rash on the trunk.

Trichoscopic findings: Perifollicular collar scaling (white arrows) is a hallmark of LP, scales from silver –white tubular structure around the emerging hair shaft.

Pili torti (red arrows) the hair shaft irregularly flattened and twisted.

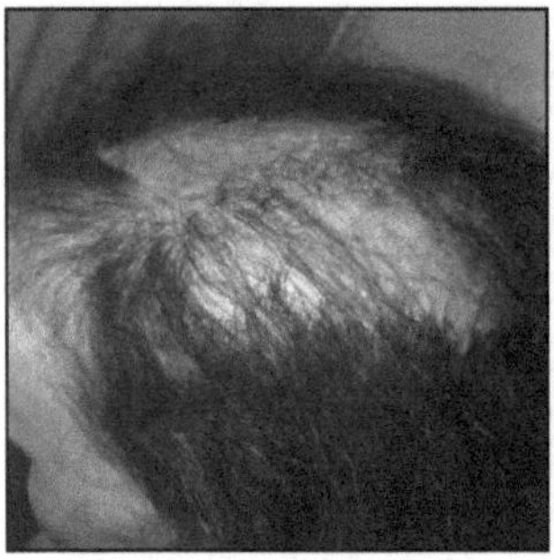
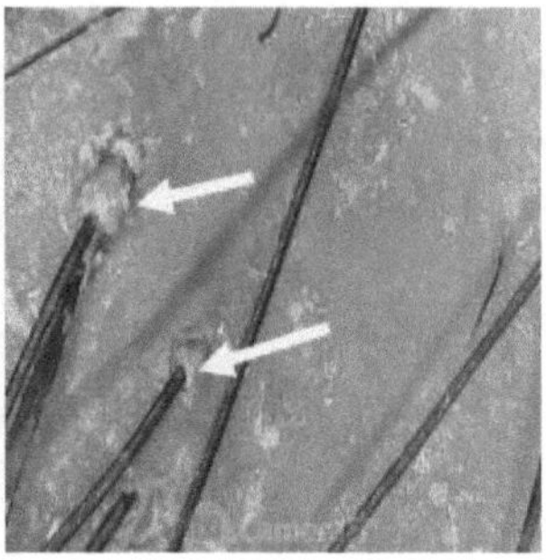
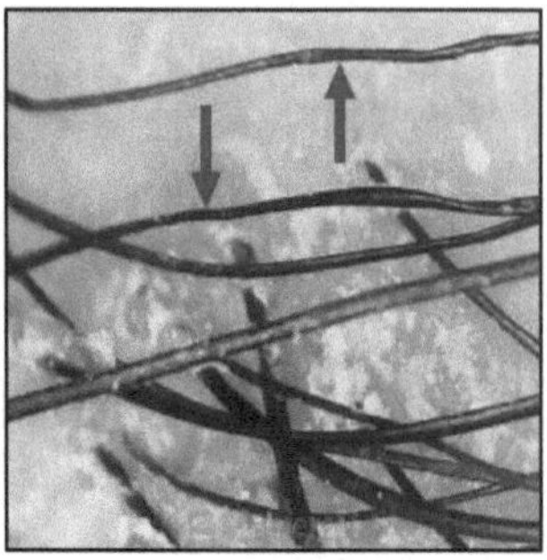

Note: pili torti

- Occasionally in normal scalp
- Common in genetic hair shaft disorders

Case- 33

A 65-years- old female patient has gradual thining and diffuse patch of hair loss on the scalp for 10 years. Trichoscopic findings: In lichen planopilaris, the tufted hair (blue arrow) is walled with silver-white scales.
Two types of white dots are visible in this photo, (red arrow) shows pinpoint white dots corresponds to eccrine sweat gland and follicular openings on sun – exposed scalp.
Large white irregular dots with bunt borders with tendency to become confluent (yellow arrow) corresponds to follicular fibrosis.

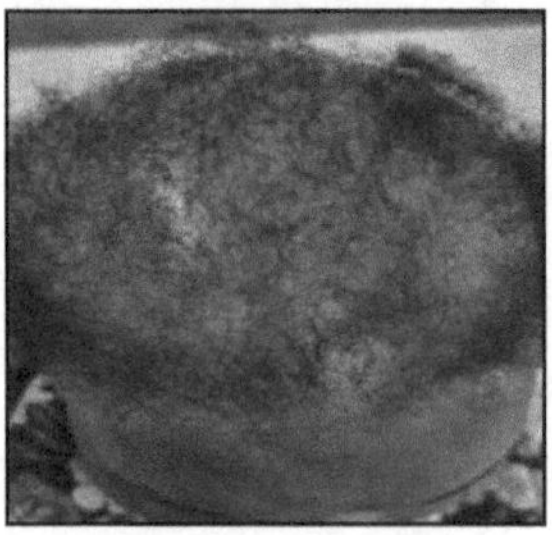
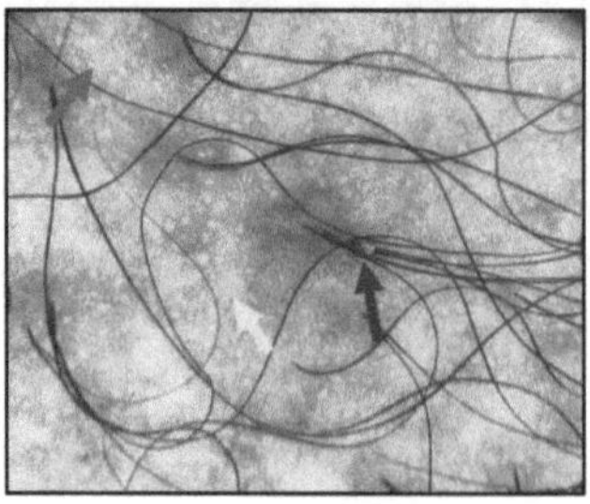

Frontal fibrosing Alopecia:

The disease is characterized clinically by slowly progressive symmetric hairline recession in the frontotemporal and /or frontoparietal region.

Trichoscopic features:

- Absence of vellus hairs.
- Lonely terminal hair is a centimeter long and may be accompanied by perifollicular scales.
- Perifollicular erythema is an indicator of the active stage.
- Peripilar casts.
- Red dots& gray or grayish dots with advanced FF.
- The eyebrow area rarely shows features of fibrosis with total loss of follicles.

Case- 34

A 55-years- old female- patient has gradual bitemporal and frontal hair line recession with diffuse hair thining and eye brows alopecia for 3 years. Trichoscopic findings: Background color is ivory pink, perifollicular erythema and scaling (white arrow), red dots (yellow arrows), elongated linear blood vessels (blue arrow).

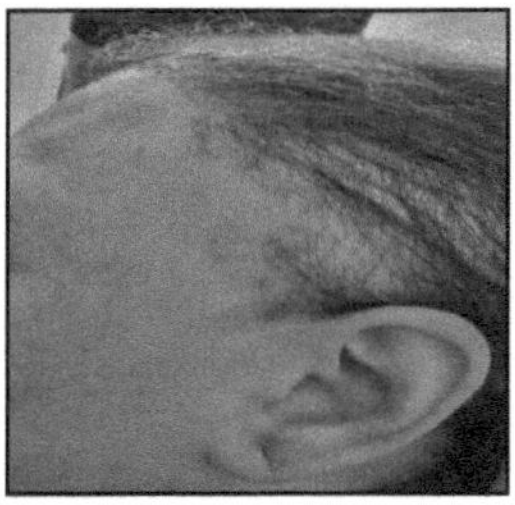

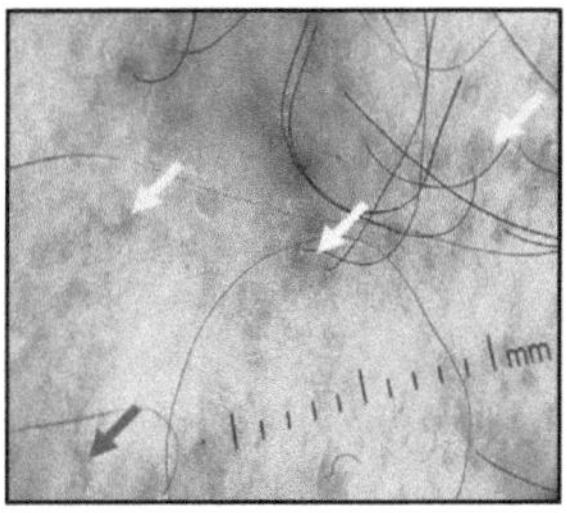

Case- 35

A 52-years- old female patient presented with baldness on frontal hair line with emerging hair as dollhair patteren for one year. Trichoscopic findings: Prifollicular scaling (yellow arrows), white dots (red arrow), lonely hair (blue arrow).

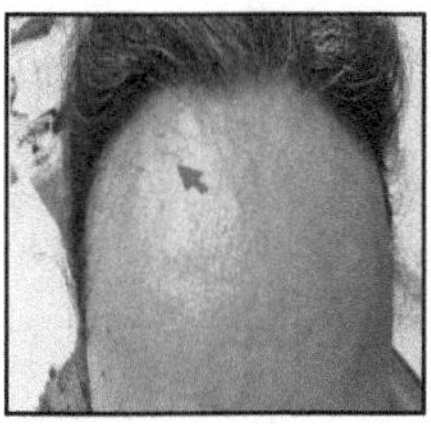

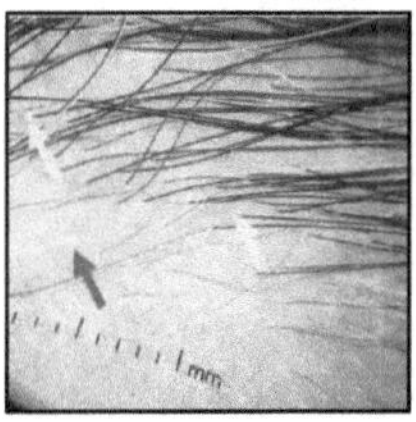

Case- 36

A 57-years- old female patient, she has clinical presentation of FFA
Eye brows trichoscopy shows:up right regrowing hairs (blue arrows) in different directions,and red dots (red arrows).

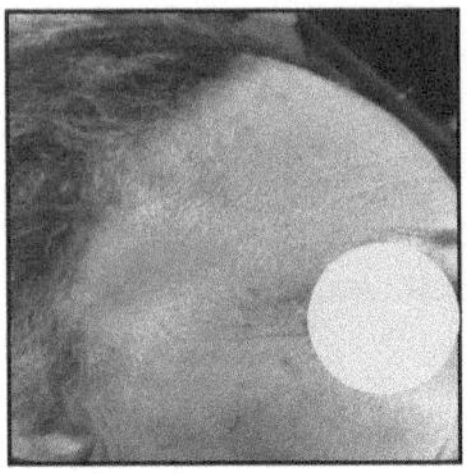
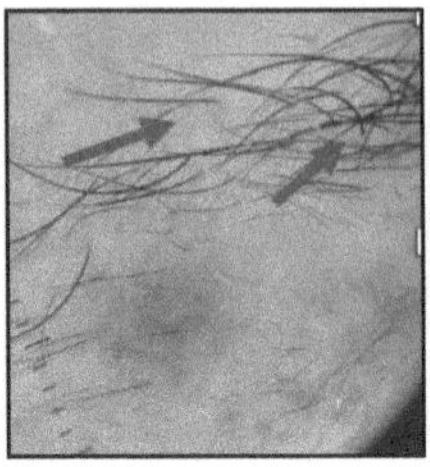
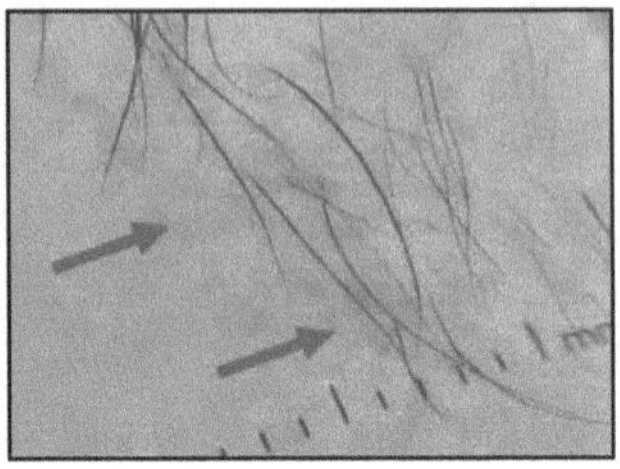

Pseudopelade of Brocq

Clinically characterized by asymptomatic, non-inflammatory white or porcelain – white, small oval/ round, reticulate, or large, irregular patches located in the central scalp area.

The distribution of alopecia patches in pseudopelade of Brocq may imitate footprints in the snow.

Trichoscopic features:

- No white dots observed.
- No follicular openings.
- Smooth white area.
- Occasionally, dystrophic hairs are found at the periphery of the lesion.
- No features indicate any type of other cicatricial alopecia (desert space).

Case- 37

A 40-years- old female- patient has gradual pogressive small patches of hair that s coalese together on vertex& parietal and frontal scalp for four years, had not history of any inflammation or scaling. Trichoscopic findings: Multifocal complete loss of the follicular ostia (red arrow), no sign of inflammation-desert space like.

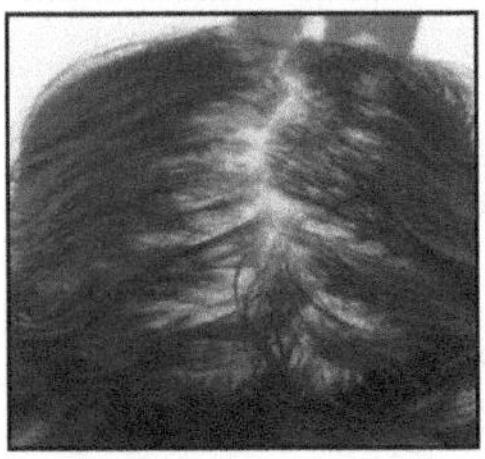
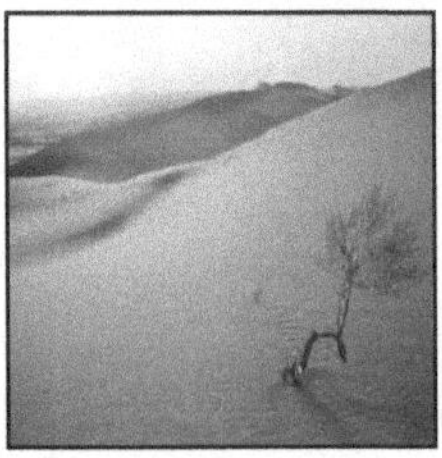
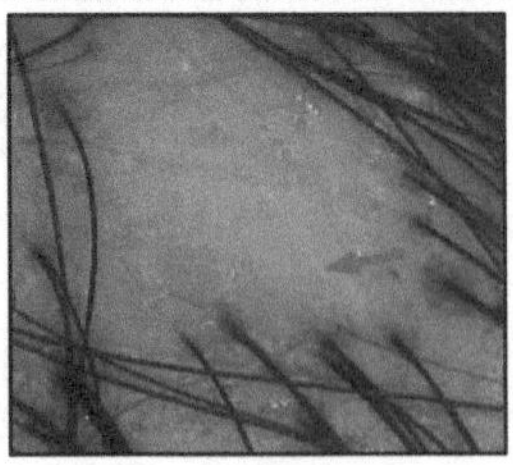

Discoid lupus erythematosus

Cicatricial alopecia is associated with active inflammatory lesions, atrophy, and telangiectasia. Present as mottled dyspigmentation, which is usually seen on the vertex and occipit.

Trichoscopic features:

- Hyperkeratotic perifollicular scales like these are seen in lichen planopilaris
- Follicular plugs.
- Perifollicular and interfollicular blue-gray dots related to pigment incontinence (melanophages).
- Loss of pigment network is seen in the black scalp.

Important clue for diagnosis:

- Scattered brown-yellow dots with a double edge are typically seen in the active stage.
- Red dots mean dilated blood vessels around the follicular openings and thick a rborizing blood vessels, both of which are indications of early acute disease and good response to therapy.
- Loss of follicular openings indicates scarring alopecia.
- White patches areas of scarring.
-

Case- 38

A 48-year- male presented with multiple patches of hair loss some of them contain white scales for 3 months, he had recurrent patchy hair loss for 10 years ago.

Trichoscopic findings: Follicular keratotic plugging (blue arrow), milky white areas (red arrow), background erythema indicates recent fibrosis, red dots appear as erythematous, and polycyclic and regularly distributed (black arrow).

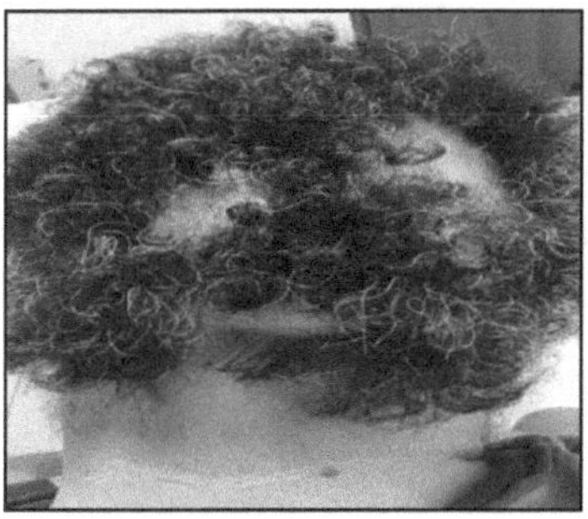

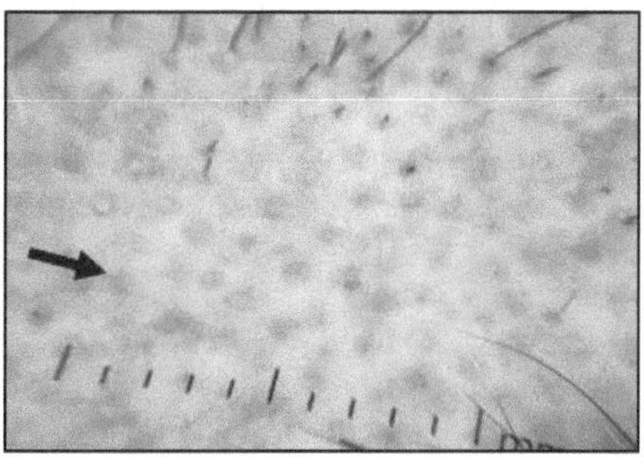

Case- 39

A 38-year- female presents with multiple patches of hair loss on scalp for 10 years, In the last 2 years diagnosed as case of SLE.

Trichoscopic findings: Keratotic plugging (black arrows).

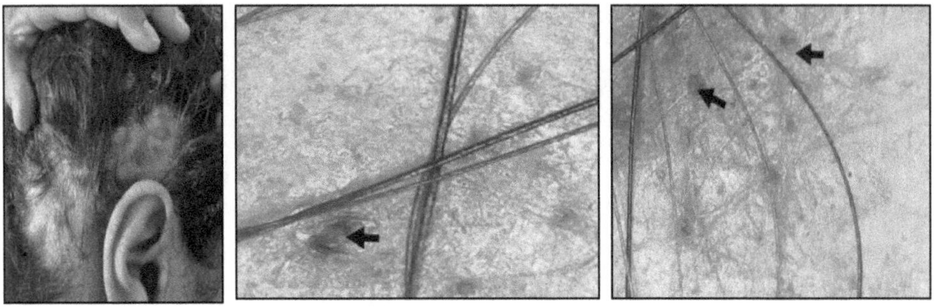

Case- 40

A 34-year- female presents with single oval patch of hair loss on the central hair line for 6 months

Trichoscopic findings: dilated blood vessels (blue arrows), and yellow dot with double edge (yellow arrow).

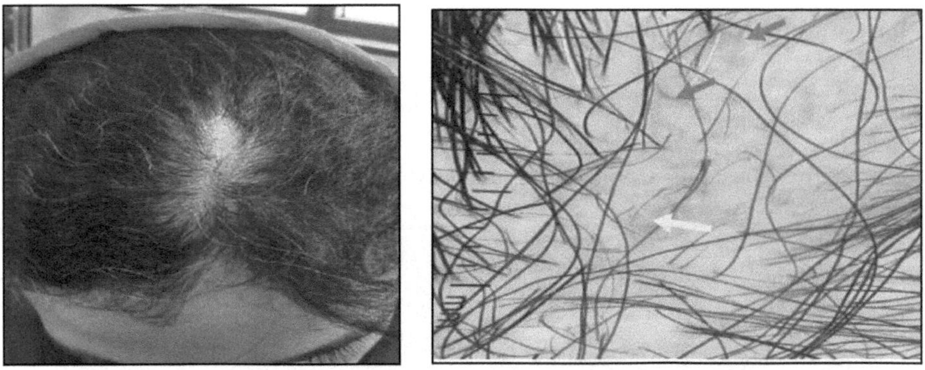

Case- 41

A 34-year- female presents with patches of hair loss on the scalp for 6 months.

Trichoscopic findings: Blue –gray dots; (black arrow), large yellow dots are sharp demarcated- double edged; follicular plugging (yellow arrow).

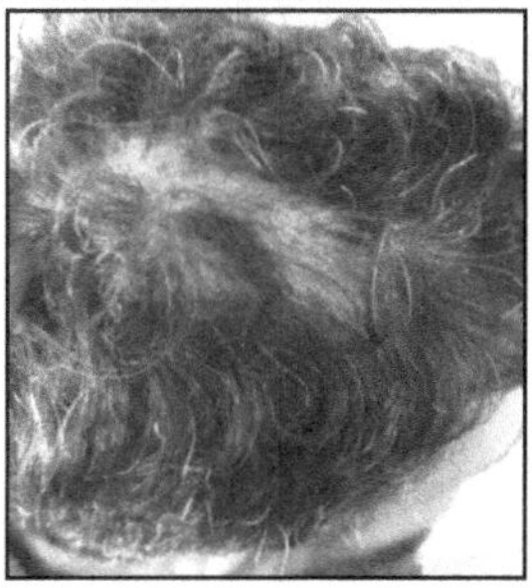

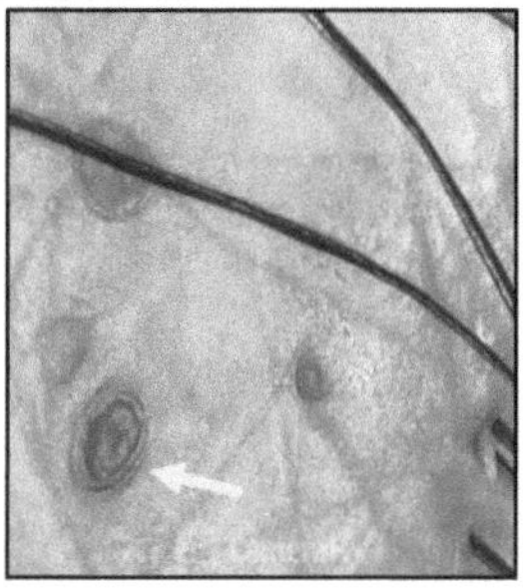

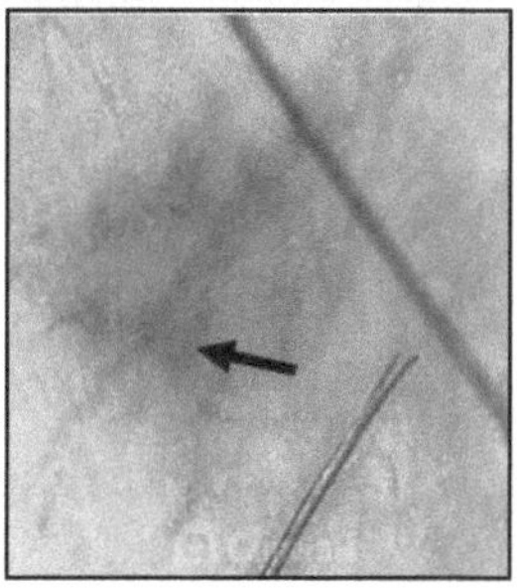

Case- 42

A 33-year- female presents multiple patches of hair loss on the scalp for 10 months.

Trichoscopic findings:

- Scattered brown discoloration (black arrows), this feature observed in active DLE lesions .
- Brown-yellow dots (yellow arrows) are bigger and darker than those seen in AA.
- Thick arborizing blood vessels (blue arrows) are thicker than an average hair shaft.

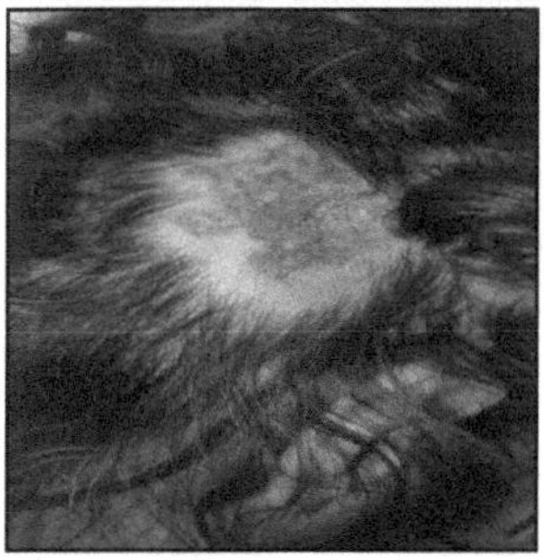

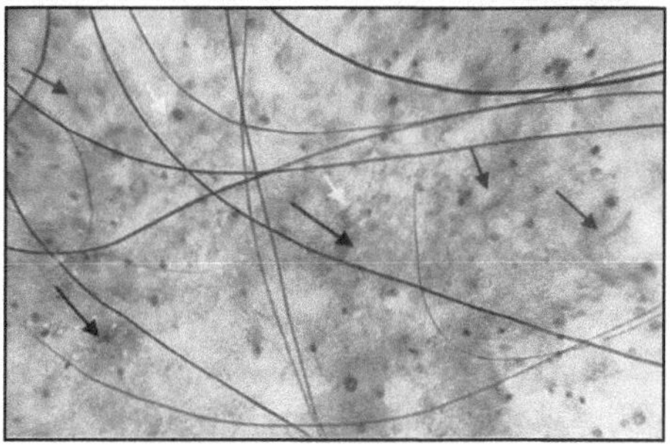

Note:
The trichoscopic characteristics of DLE depend on disease duration and activity.

Central Centrifugal Scarring Alopecia

Central centrifugal cicatricial alopecia is the most common form of scarring hair loss seen in black women. Many factors are incorporated in the pathogenesis of CCCA, including genetic factors and hair styling practices.

Trichoscopic features:

- Peripilar whitish halo has been seen in early and late stage CCCA, corresponding to the lamellar fibrosis surrounding the hair follicle, the outer root sheath
- Steak-like brown blotches, broken hairs, and dark peripilar halo are considered particular features of CCCA
- Pinpoint white dots
- Honeycomb pigmentation
- Scaling

Case- 43

A 58-year- female presents with gradual hair loss as large patch of on frontal& vertex for 5 years.

Trichoscopic findings:

- Dark peripilar halo (black arrow).
- Disrupted pigmented network (red arrow).
- Loss of follicular openings (yellow arrow).

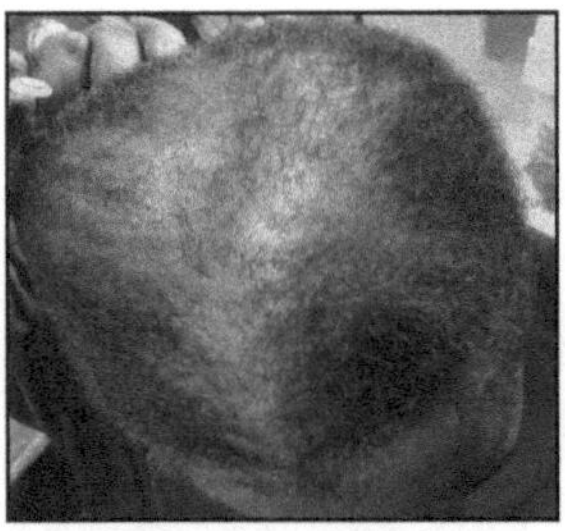
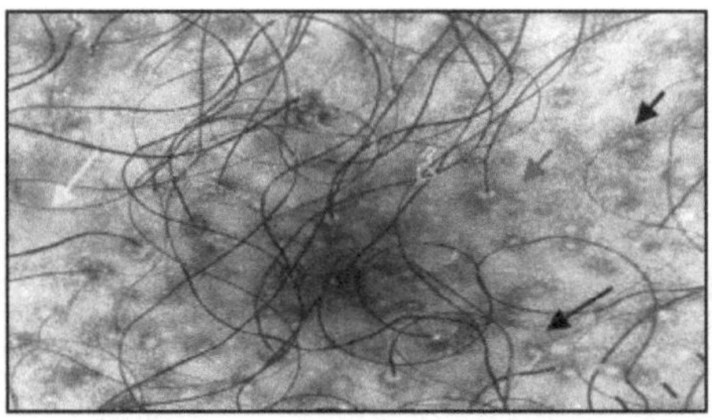

Keratosis Follicularis Spinulosa Decalvans

Inherited skin and scalp condition, mostly seen in men, presented with scarring alopecia affecting the scalp and eyebrows.

Case- 44

A 19-year- old male presented to us complaining of itchy scaly scalp and eyebrows with gradual hair loss for 5 years, associated with facial erythema and generalized popular scaly lesions.

Trichoscopic findings

- Perifollicular whitish scales (red arrow).
- Single hair perifollicular unit (yellow arrow).
- Perifollicular erythematous violaceous halo (blue arrows).

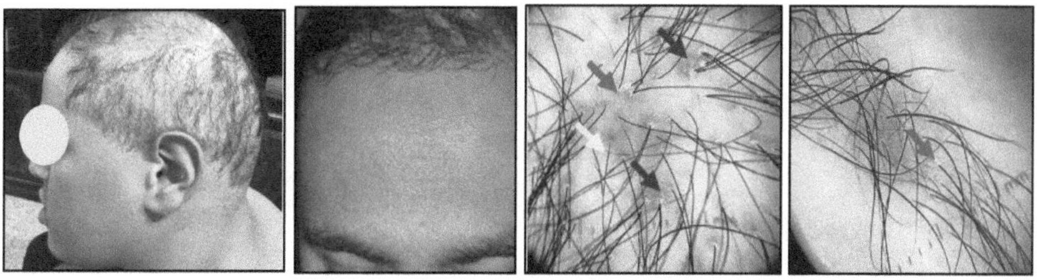

Note:
Scarring alopecia

- Handlebar sign: showing curved hair attached to the skin on both ends (green arrow).
- White area (possibly) indicating fibrosis and scaling, underlying linear bluish pigmentation indicating the buried hair shaft (red arrow).

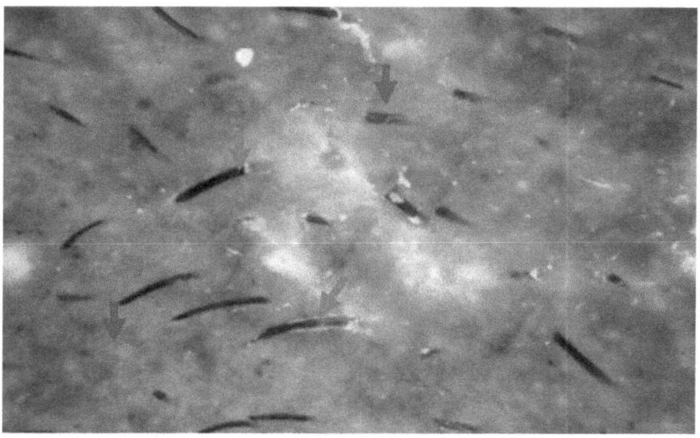

Trichoscopic features of common types of scarring alopecia

LPP	FFA	DLE
Intense perifollicular scaling, tubular structures	Few perifollicular scaling	Follicular keratotic plugging
Violaceous interfollicular areas	Perifollicular erythema	Mottled dyschromia
White dots	Single hair follicular units at the scalp margin	Thin and radial arborizing vessels that emerge from yellow dots (red spider in yellow dot)
Small hair tufts	Absence of vellus hair	Arborizing blood vessels at the periphery of the lesion
Blue-gray dots	Pale gray/ red dots on the lateral eyebrows	Follicular dots

Folliculitis Decalvans

FD is a form of cicatricial alopecia due to neutrophilic inflammation.

Key trichoscopic signs:

- Follicular pustules.
- Tufted hairs (multiple hairs that emerged from a single dilated opening are 6 or more in number) due to intense inflammation surrounding the follicular openings, it is very characteristic, but it is not specific.
- Perifollicular hyperplasia arranged in a starburst pattern (white arrow), which is an indication of disease progression.

Note:
Starburst appears due to dermal fibrosis with loss of elastic fibers may be responsible for the radiating undulatory appearance.

- Tubular like scales with collar –like widening at the distal end present in over 60% of patients.
- Crusts yellow to hemorrhagic.
- Red strawberry ice cream areas.
- Loss of follicular opening& white dots indicate disease fibrotic changes.

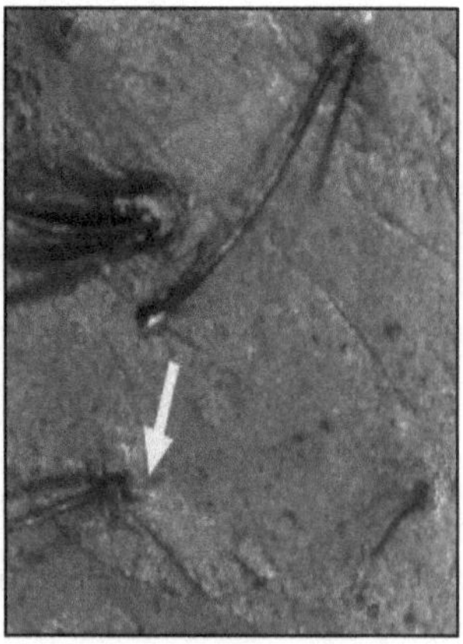

Case- 45

A 29-years old male patient presented with indurated patch of hair loss involves the vertex and occipital area of the scalp.

Trichoscopic findings

Starburst hyperplasia (red arrow), surrounding doll like tufted hairs (yellow arrow), follicular opening with eight hairs, prominent perifollicular scaling (blue arrow), yellow crusts and hemorrhagic crusts (black arrow).

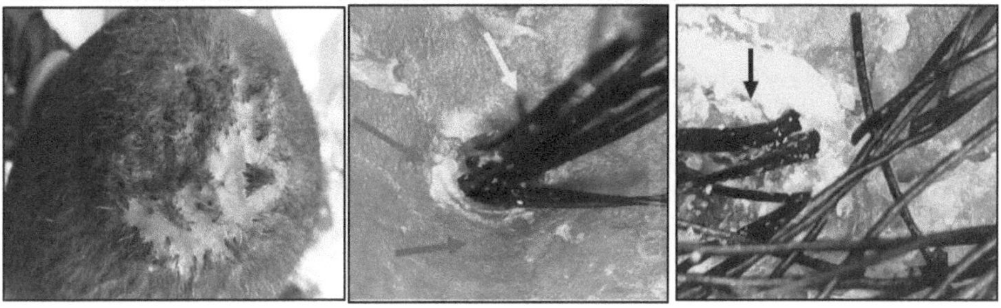

Case- 46

A 35-year- male patient has erythematous scarring plaques, crustation and purulent area is visible on the scalp for 3years.

Trichoscopic findings

- White Tubular like scales with collar (red arrow).
- Yellow perifollicular discoloration with visible plugging (yellow arrow)

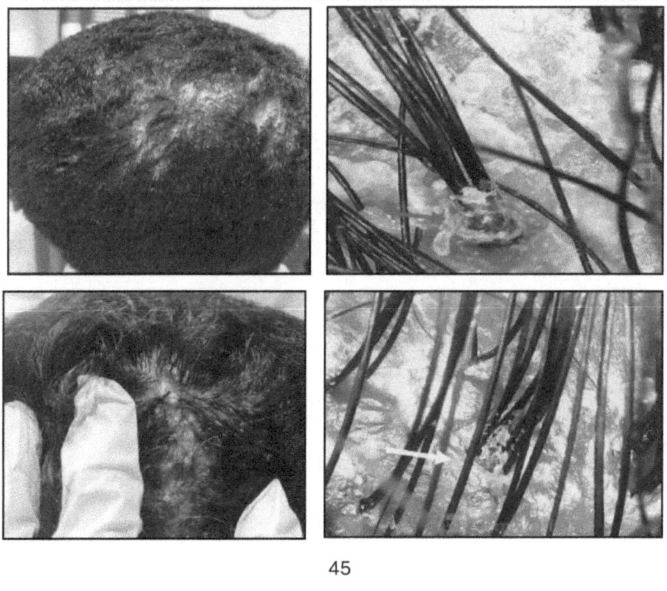

Dissecting cellulitis

dissecting folliculitis, perifolliculitis capitus abscedens et suffodiens.

DS is a chronic progressive, inflammatory disease characterized by perifollicular pustules, nodules, and abscesses with interconnecting sinus tracts. Nodules are firm or fluctuant, and purulent material that evolves into scarring alopecia.
Together with acne conglobata, hidradenitis suppurative, and pilonidal cysts, the disease forms a syndrome called follicular occlusion tetrad.

Trichoscopic features of the active stage:

- Yellow structureless areas; these areas correspond to dense neutrophilic dermal infiltrates on histopathology.
- Yellow dots 3D soap bubble dots with or without hair shafts.
- Black dots pinpoint like vessels with a whitish halo.
- Cutaneous clefts with emerging hairs.
- Hair tufts.

Case- 47

A 38-years-old female presents painful multiple pustules & nodules on vertex for 2 months, recurrent nodules and abscess collection on axilla and anal region was surgically treated for the past 3 years.
Trichoscopic findings: Yellow dots appearing as large 3 D soap bubbles (red arrow) imposed over dark dystrophic hairs.

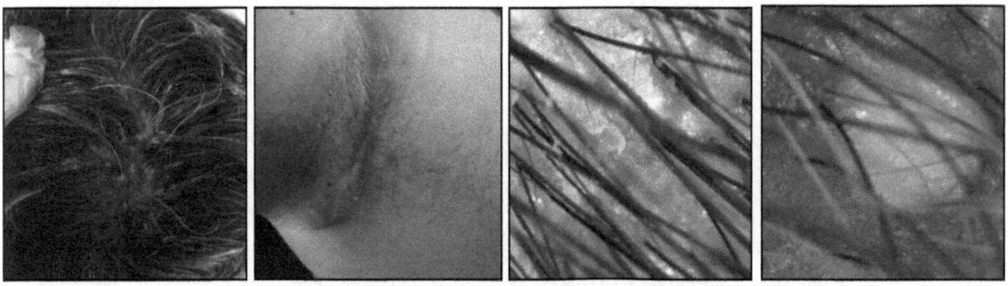

Note:
Differential diagnosis of DS:

- Folliculitis decalvans
- Acne keloidalis nuchae folliculotropic mycosis fungoides
- Alopecia mucinosa
- Tinea capitus

Acne Keloidalis Nuchae (synonymous folliculitis keloidalis)

It is unusual for inflammation of the hair follicle units on the nape of the neck to proceed to keloid-like scarring, which is more common in dark –skinned people than in whites.

Trichoscopy:
Multiple hair shafts emerging from a single follicular opening.

Case- 48

A 33-year-old man with 3years history of small erythematous papules and pustules on the nape of the neck.

Trichoscopy features:

- Perifollicular pustules and white halo surrounding hair follicles (red arrow).
- Dilated follicular ostia filled with keratin associated black dots (yellow arrow).
- Perifollicular pustules and tufted hairs (blue arrow).

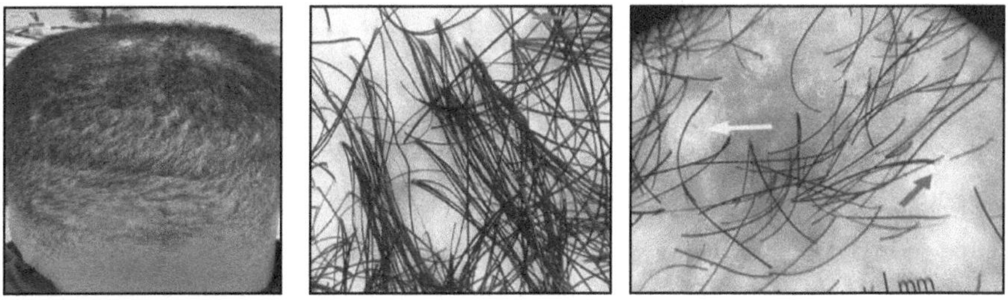

Tufted hairs present in:

- Folliculitis decalvans (very frequent)
- Lichen planopilaris (frequent)
- Discoid lupus erythematosus (rare)
- Central centrifugal cicatricial alopecia (rare)
- Acne keloidalis (rare)
- Dissecting cellulitis
- Tinea capitus
- Pemphigus
- Hair transplantation
- Drugs: epidermal growth factor receptor.

Epidermal scaling

I. Dandruff

It is generally caused by fungi known as Malassezia Globosa, which feed on sebum secretion on the scalp in extreme situations of excess oil secretion, growing fungi, and break down sebum into oleic acid. If your body reacts to this, it leads to severe itching & erythema, and white scales of dead epidermal cells.

II. Diffuse:

- Normal
- Psoriasis-white
- Seborrheic dermatitis- yellow
- Discoid lupus erythematosus-white

III. Perifollicular:

- Lichen planopilaris- tubular /white
- Frontal fibrosing alopecia-white
- Folliculitis decalvans-yellow-collar like

3. Inflammatory scalp disorders

Psoriasis and seborrheic dermatitis are both erythematosquamous dermatoses that can involve the scalp. Trichoscopy may help to differentiate scalp psoriasis and seborrheic dermatitis, where videodermoscopy is used for better vascular images than handheld dermoscopy.

3.1 Psoriasis

Atypical red vessels, red dots and globules, coiled vessels, and twisted red loops

Structureless red areas and hidden hairs.

3.2 Seborrheic dermatitis

Arborizing vessels are typical features that appear to be increased compared with healthy controls, with the absence of red dots and globules.

Note:

- Signet ring shape (SRV) is thought to be formed by tortuous glomerular vessel and its elongated and dilated annular ring-shaped vessel. Considered as a specific sign for these dermatoses when compared with other alopecia
- SRVsign detected more common in psoriasis.
- Hidden hairs: pilosebaseous unit with proximal hair shaft appears as hidden hair under a white – grey epidermal proliferation
- Comma vessels are considered as specific sign for seborrheic dermatitis

Case- 49

A 10-year- old boy presented with single large scaly patch on erythematous background on the scalp and hyperkeratotic small plaques on extensor extremities for 4 months.

Trichoscopic findings: Silver –white scaling; red arrow, regular distributed dotted (glomerular) vessels (blue arrow), signet ring vessels (yellow arrow), hidden hair (green arrow).

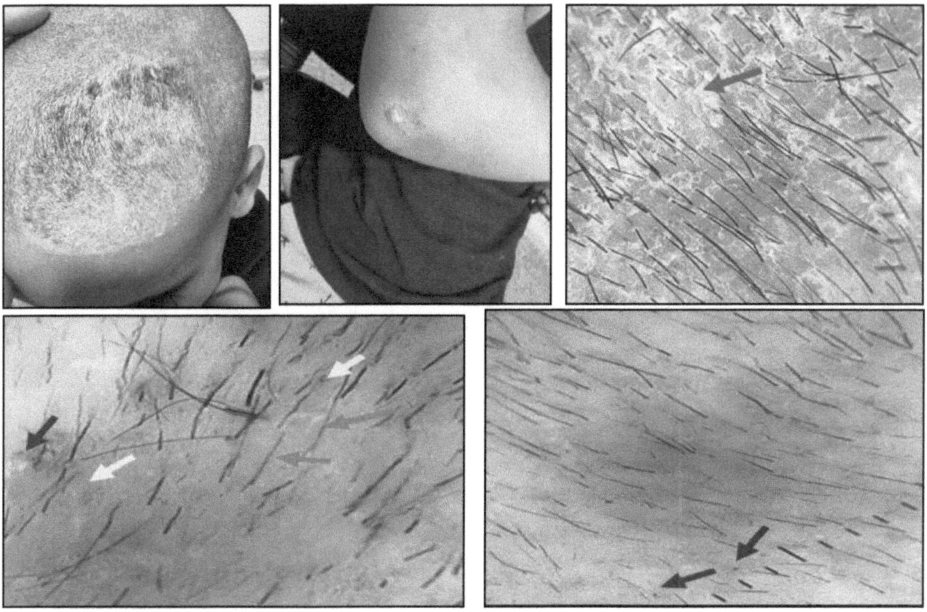

Case- 50

A 12-year-girl presents with recurrent erythematous scaly plaque on the nape on neck, she has positive family history of psoriasis.

Trichoscopic findings: White scaling; blue arrow, twisted red loops arranged in homogenous pattern on light erythematous background; yellow arrows.

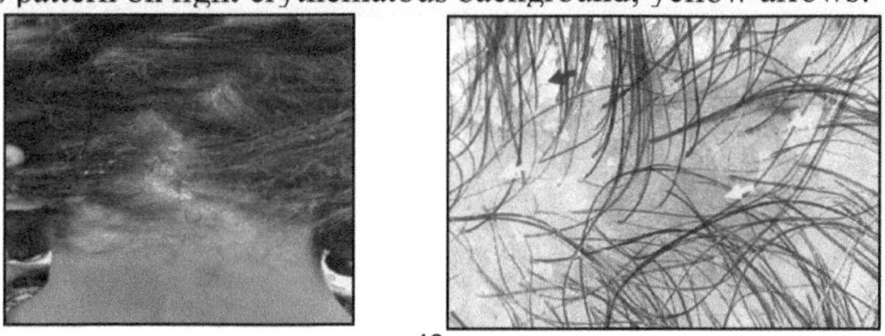

Case- 51

A 22-year-male patient has oily skin presents greasy scales on scalp, eyebrows, sides of the nose, and behind the ears.
Trichoscopic findings: Thin arborizing vessels are observed (white arrows).

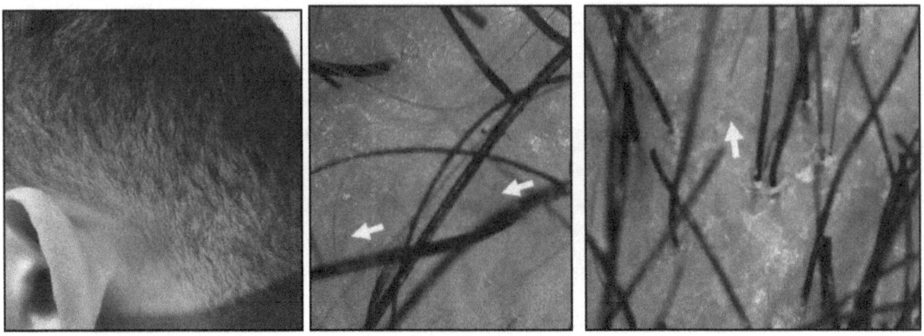

4. Autoimmune bullous disease

Pemphigus foliaceous: PF is characterized immunologically by the presence of circulating and in vivo bound antibodies against desmoglein 1 and 3.

The estimated incidence of scalp involvement in pemphigus ranges from 5 to 50%.

Case- 52

A 58-year-old female presented p with longstanding pemphigus foliaceous confirmed on clinical and histopathological study, she has resistant scalp pemphigus lesions to therapy were given. On physical examination of the scalp lesions: whitish& yellowish scales on erythematous base and decreased hair density on frontal –vertex and parietal regions.

Trichoscopic findings: Dotted vessels with whitish halo (blue arrows), multiple yellow dots pierced by hair shafts with whitish halo, fried-egg sign (red arrows) and whitish lamellar scales with protruding edge correspond to partly detached elements of the epidermis (black arrow).

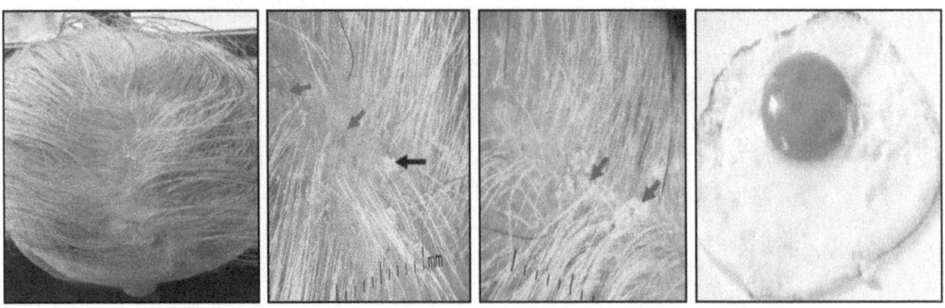

5. Pediatric Hair Disorders

Hair loss in early childhood represents a broad differential diagnosis that can be a diagnostic and therapeutic challenge. It is important to consider the diagnosis of a genetic hair disorder. Genetic hair disorders are a large group of inherited disorders, many of which are rare.

5.1 Diffuse Alopecia Areata:

- Also known as alopecia areata incognito, which is a very rare form of AA, it can affect both sexes at any age, causing excessive hair shedding and thinning of the entire scalp, and they have a positive pulling test within months.
- Laboratory workup should be performed to identify treatable causes such as serum ferritin, zinc, and vitamin D, TSH, LFT, RFT, and ANA.
- Commonly misdiagnosed as telogen effluvium, loose anagen hair syndrome, and trichotellomania.

Case- 53

A 4-years –female child presented with diffuse hair loss from scalp and eyebrows for 2 months which was preceded by high fever due to upper respiratory infection, she has positive family history for alopecia areata. Clinically there is diffuse alopecia with lack of characteristic patches of AA.

Trichoscopic pictures shows broken hair; black arrow, multiple yellow dots (green arrow), black dots (yellow arrow), elbow hair (red arrow).

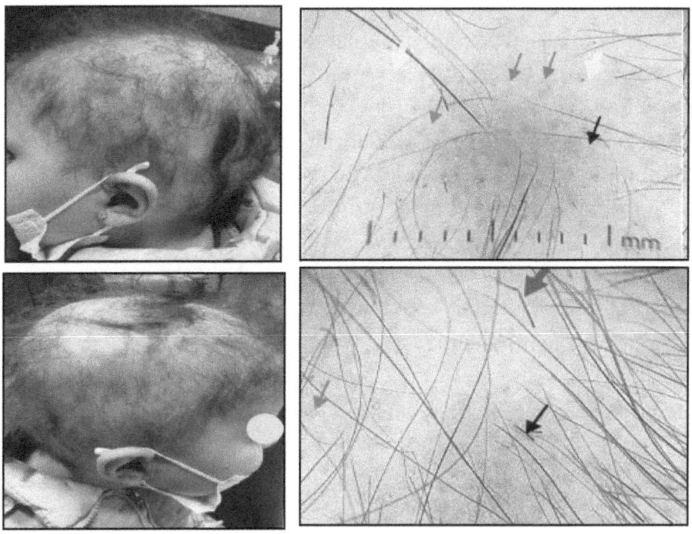

5.2 Telogan Effluvium (TE)

It is a diffuse cyclic hair loss; it is transitory episodes of reversible diffuse hair shedding.

Case- 54

A 3-years – old boy his parents present him with sudden diffuse hair loss from scalp for 3months. The child had history of gastroenteritis before hair shedding and the results of laboratory tests were very low serum ferritin & vitamin D levels.

Trichoscopy examination shows decreased total hair count and increased single hair follicular unit (black arrows), dirt's (red arrows).

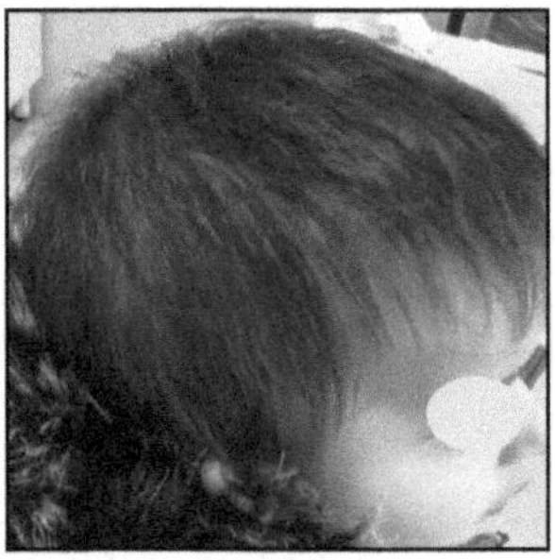

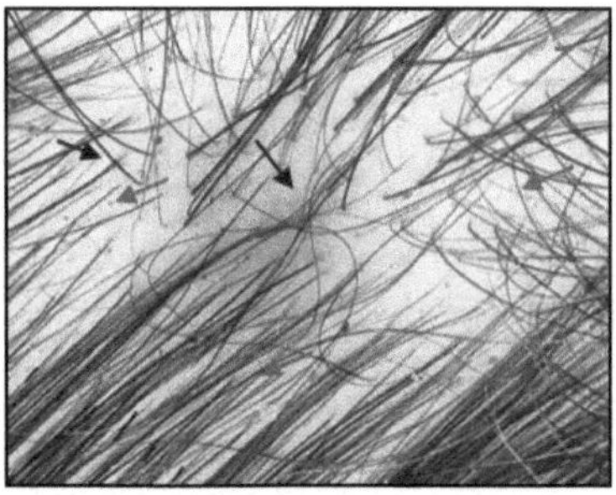

5.3 Sebaceous Nevus

- Also called nevus sebaceous of Jadasson or organoid, characterized by hyperplasia of the epidermis, immature hair follicles, and sebaceous and apocrine glands.
- Nevus sebaceous is a type of epidermal nevus, which is also called schimmelpenning syndrome, classified as a benign hair follicle tumor
- Clinical presentation is divided into three stages: **at birth,** in childhood, it appears as a solitary hairless plaque with a waxy appearance and yellowish-orange in color. During **adolescence,** lesions become more verrucous, and **in adults**, they are commonly associated with secondary neoplasms.
- Often oval or linear in shape.

Differential diagnosis:

1. Aplasia cutis congenital
2. Juvenile xanthogranuloma
3. Epidermal nevus

Trichoscopy is an important diagnostic tool for diagnosing and monitoring nevus sebaceous to detect an early tumors change.

Case- 55

Female 12years old presented with yellowish-brown plaque on vertex since childhood. On trichoscopic examination: Brown ill-defined globular arrangement in cerebriform pattern (red arrow).

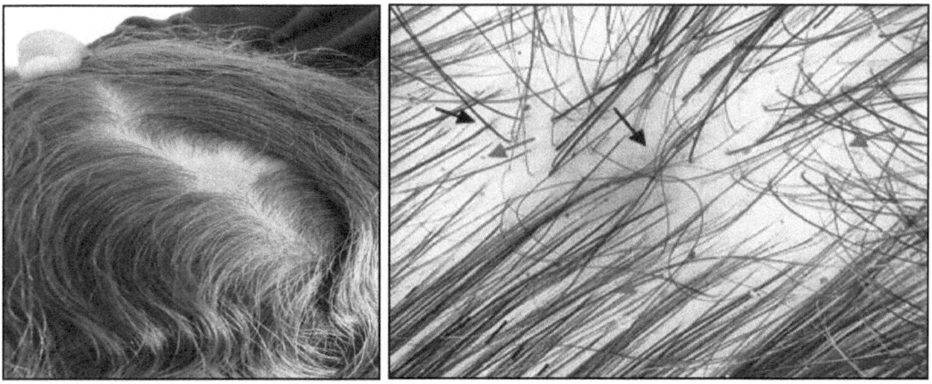

Case- 56

An 8-years- old boy presented with small yellowish-brown plaque on vertex for 3 years, on trichoscopic examination: revealed orange well defined globular structures cobblestone pattern (blue arrow).

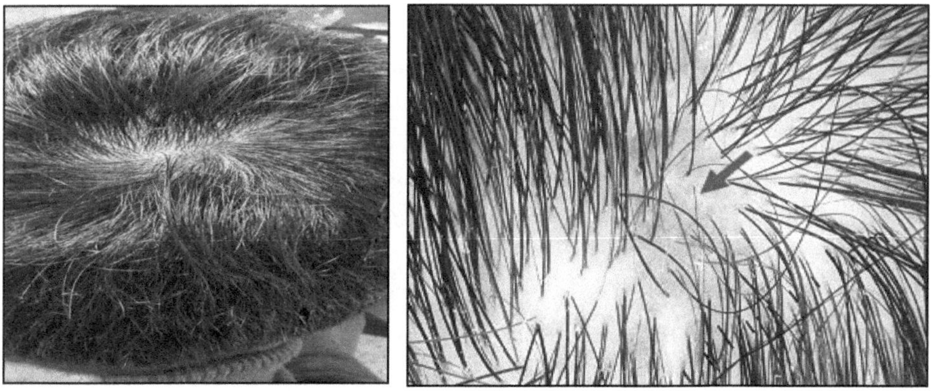

5.4 Aplasia Cutis Congenital

Rare skin defect characterized by a focal or multiple absent skin, occasionally subcutaneous tissue, since birth, although 70 to 90 percent of lesions are localized to the vertex of the scalp, it can appear on any body part.

Trichoscopic features

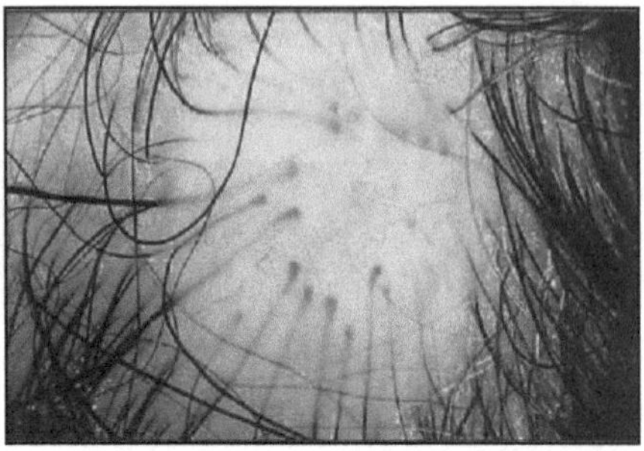

Shows a brown to bright white structureless area with the absence of follicular ostia with brown dots –peppering at the center with radially and horizontally hair shafts arranged at the periphery with visible proximal hair bulbs. A collar of hair is often seen around the defect: Skin appendage disorder.

Case- 57

A 40-days-infant, born with normal vaginal delivery, his parents described the appearance of the eroded lesions at birth that increased in size, there was no history of the similar illness in the child family. The infant was treated conservatively with topical antibiotic cream & antiseptic solution and dressing; he had no ophthalmic and neurologic findings and no specific laboratory abnormalities.

Physical examination shows fibrotic scar and alopecia on midline of the frontal& vertex scalp and small hemorrhagic crusts on vertex. The dermatological diagnosis of aplasia cutis congenital was established, based on clinical and dermoscopic findings.

Trichoscopic examination showed large plaque on frontal-vertex scalp with erythema and white background & numerous thin arborizing blood vessels, absence of follicular openings, hair bulbs with pigmented proximal ends were visible through the translucent epidermis.

Trichoscopy shows a patch of translucent skin with multiple branched blood vessels; black arrows, and hair bulbs at the margin of the defect (blue arrow), hemorrhagic crust (green arrow).

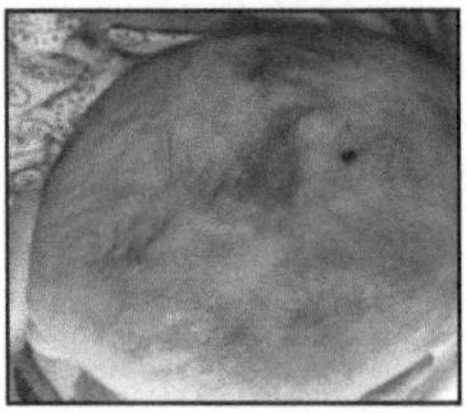

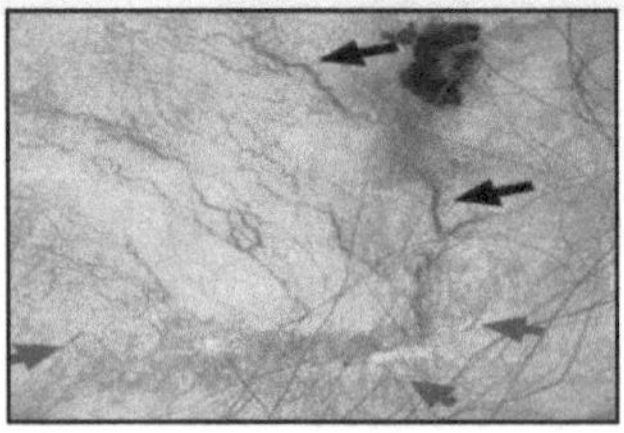

5.5 Congenital Triangular Alopecia

Also referred to as temporal triangular alopecia, it is an uncommon dermatosis of unknown etiology. A non–scarring, circumscribed, oval or triangular alopecia (the pointy aspect of the triangle points upwards to the crown), often located unilaterally in the frontotemoral region.

Differential diagnosis:

- Alopecia areata
- Trichotellomania
- Traction alopecia
- Congenital aplasia cutis

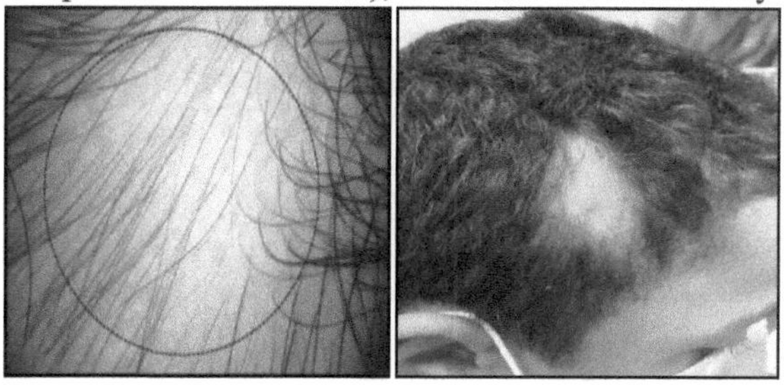

Trichoscopic features of congenital triangular alopecia: clustered short vellus hairs without other specific findings (dotted circle).

Case- 58

A16-years-old female complaining of patchy hair did not grow with the time since childhood. On physical examination: yellow-brown discolored oval patch of alopecia on temporal region. Trichoscopic examination reveals few vellus hair (blue arrows).

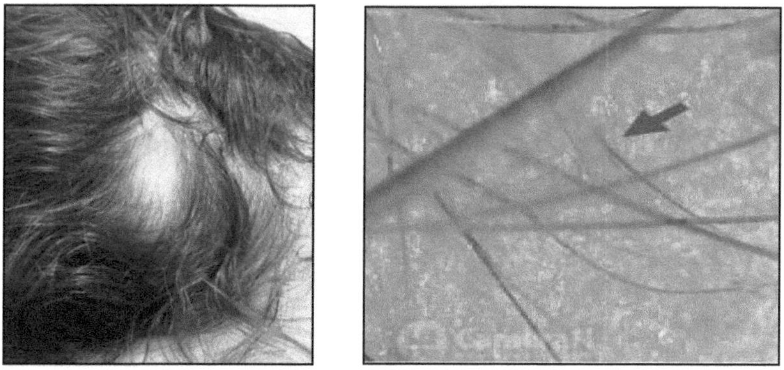

5.6 Traumatic Alopecia

Results from the forceful extraction of hair, traction, or other physical trauma. Including pressure, such as occurs in neonates who develop caput succedaneum with a scalp ring from birth trauma or use of suction at delivery, and as is seen on the occiput of infants who lie on their backs, prolonged bed rest in one position.

Case- 59

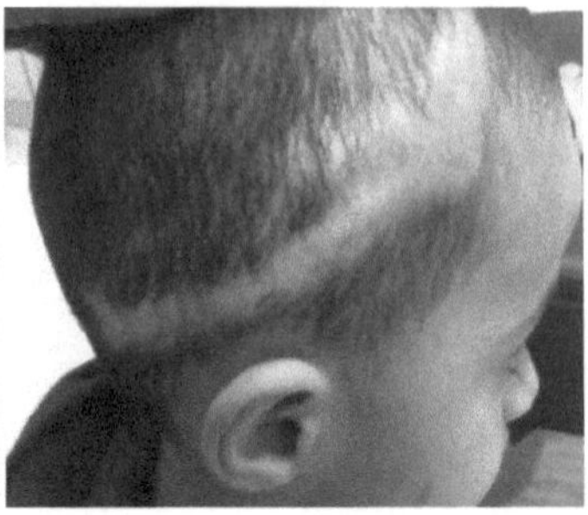

A 3-year-boy presented with scarring hair loss in linear occipital region extending to the temporo-parietal region bilaterally, the diagnosis of traumatic alopecia was made based on history of prolonged, difficult labor with vacuum- assisted delivery.

Case- 60

A boy of 9 months of age presented with hair loss in linear occipital region extending to the parietal region bilaterally, diminished hair has been noticed a few weeks after their birth through normal vaginal delivery without any assistant machine or acquired trauma. Has normal hair pull test, Clinical diagnosis of pressure alopecia was made.
On trichoscopic examination shows vellus hairs (blue arrow) without any other changes like scales or any colored dots or exclamation marks.

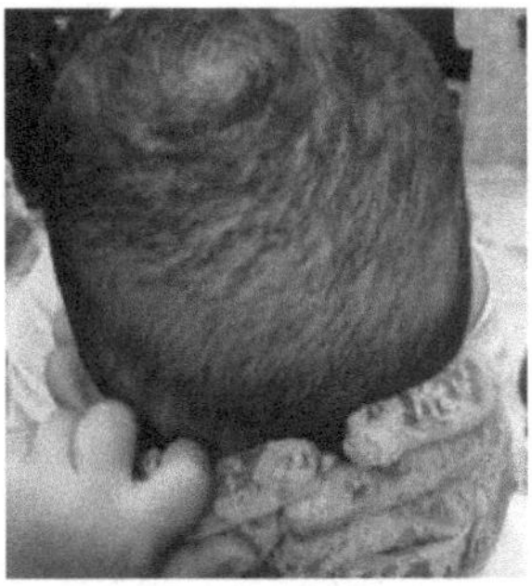

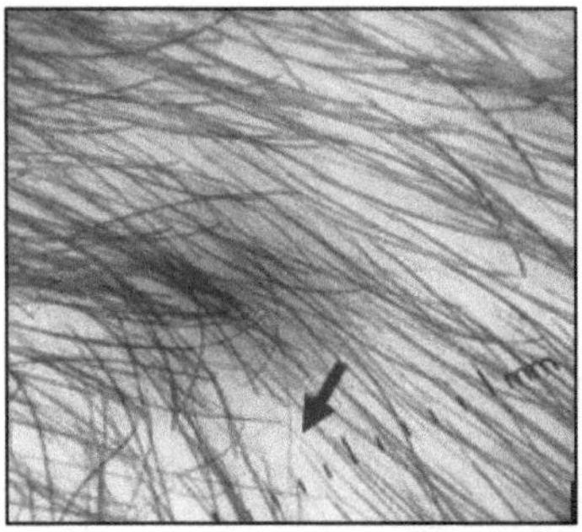

5.7 Androgenetic Alopecia

Pediatric AGA diagnosis depends on the pattern of hair loss in relation to positive family history and atypical trichoscopy.

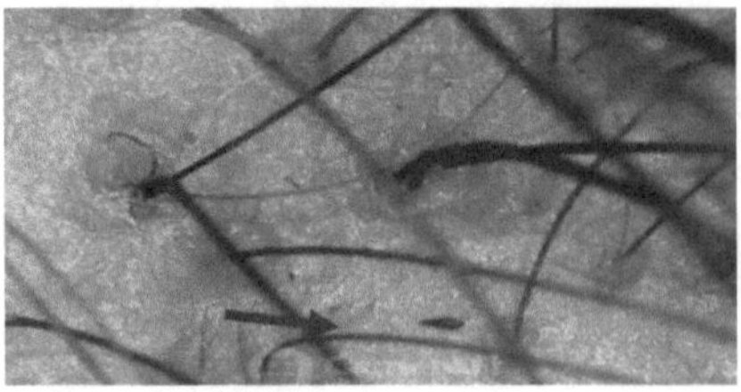

AGA has been observed as early as 6 years of age. Although the prevalence of the metabolic syndrome is increased in patients with early-onset androgenetic alopecia.

Trichoscopic examination: more than 20% of thin hairs (hair diameter variability), follicular unit with single hair shaft, yellow dots (blue arrow), perifollicular discoloration (red arrow), and an increase in the number of villus hair.

Case- 61

A 15-years –female presented with decrease hair density and hair thinning gradually over last 3 years, she has strong family history of androgenetic alopecia

On clinical examination: widen central parting.

Trichoscopy findings:

- Variation in number of hairs in each follicular unit, (white arrows).
- Perifollicular brown halo (red arrow), vellus hair (yellow arrows).

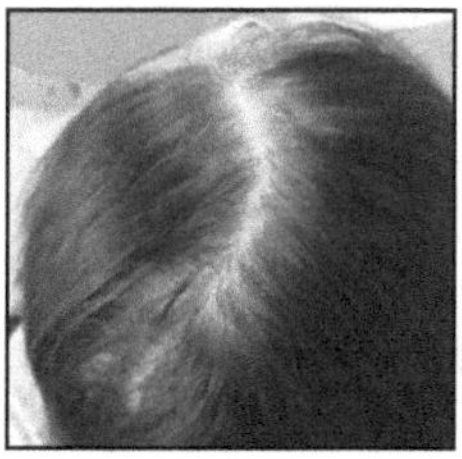

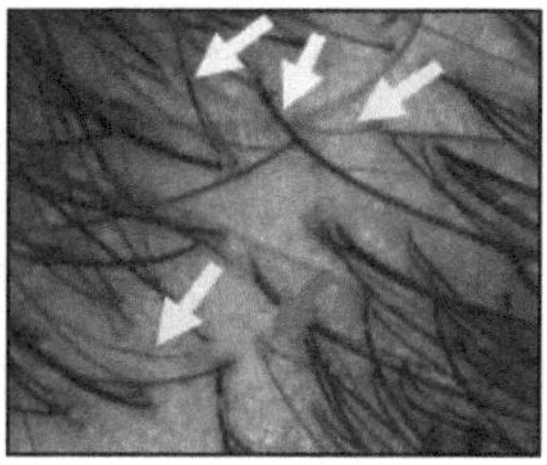

6. Hair Shaft Disorders

Steps in the diagnosis of hair shaft disorders:

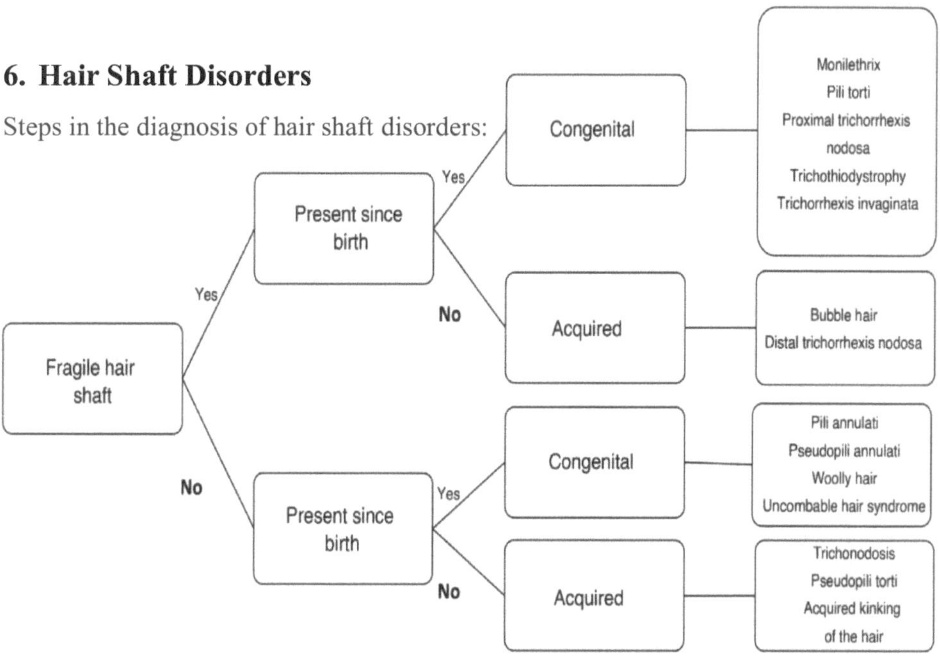

Loose Anagen Hair Syndrome

- Characterized by easy and pain-free detachment of anagen-staged hairs from the scalp.
- Ages of 2 and 8 it is especially observed in females.
- Children with light colored hair.
- Occurring as isolated cases but rarely in association with hereditary and developmental disorders.
- Presumed to be due to dis-adhesion or weak adhesion between the hair cuticale and inner root sheath in the anagen stage, and they have a characteristic rippled or ruffled, sawtooth (rumpled sock appearance) is not able to grow to a long length.

Case- 62

A 7-year- old girl child presented with diffuse scalp hair thinning & easily detached, the parents reported inability of hair to growing in length since birth, her sister and brother they have of the same complaint. Eyebrows, eyelashes, nails, and eyes were normal.

Scalp examination and trichoscopic findings: revealed diffuse thin, Pseudomonilithrix irregular spaced nodes, the nodes are wider than the normal shafts, occurring near the site of overlap the hairs.

Microscopic examination:

(a) Plucked hair with dark pigmented bulb (red arrow), absence of the inner root sheath and saw tooted and baggy stocking appearance of the cutical.

(b) Pseudomonilethrix (Black arrows).

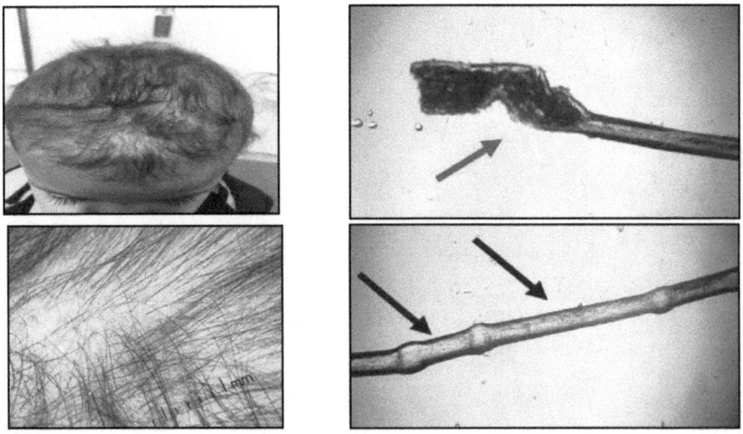

Note:

- The differential diagnosis: Trichotellomania, Alopecia areata or Telogen effluvium
- Pull hair test: painless extraction was positive of anagen hair. The diagnosis made on the history &clinical presentation and microscopic examination.

Pseudomonilethrix

Rectangular indentation on one side of the hair shaft must be differentiated from irregular fusiform narrowing of Pol Pinkus constriction.

In this case, pseudomonilithrix either acquired or iatrogenic, it is caused by trauma to the hair during the preparation (for example, compression by forceps during traction applied or pressing of the hairs between glass slides).

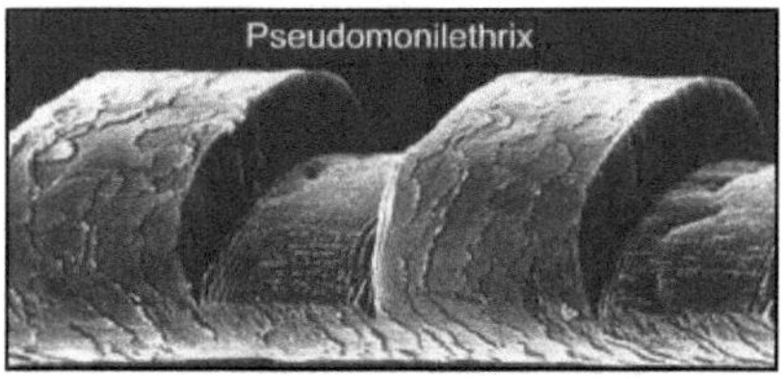

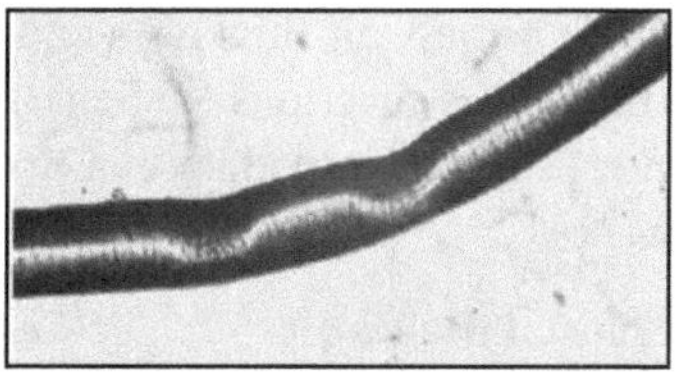

Short Anagen Hair Syndrome

It is a condition where hair does not grow beyond a short length, due to an unusually short duration of active hair growth (anagen phase), and an increased number of telogen hairs. Most cases are associated with fine blond hair.

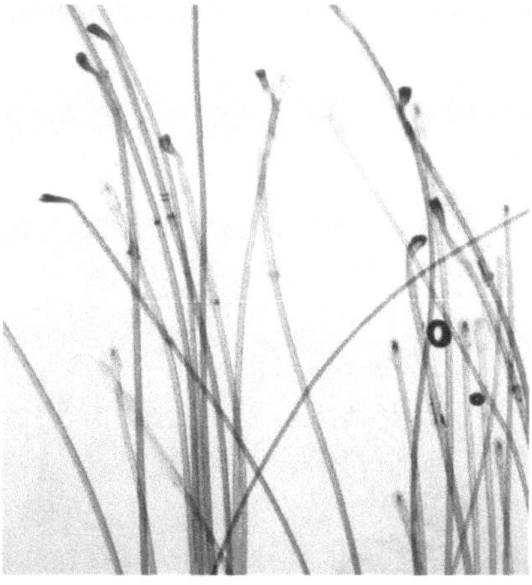

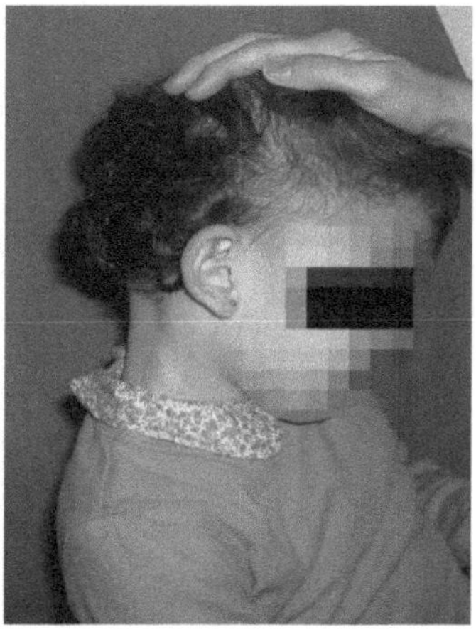

Hair shaft disorders with hair fragility

1) Monilethrix:

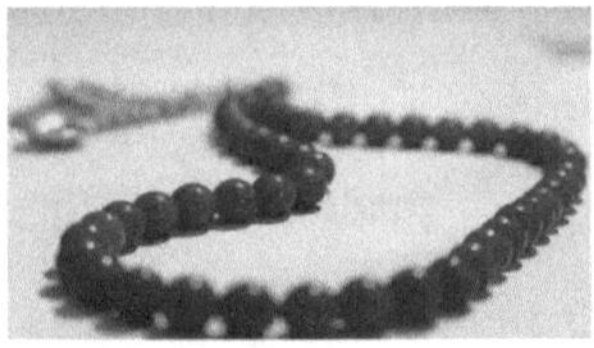

- The term monilethrix comes from monile (Latin) and thrix Greek), meaning necklace and hair, respectively.
- Monilethrix is a rare disorder of beaded hair shaft structure that breaks off at the thinner parts between the beads. It presents with hair fragility and patchy alopecia.
- Monilethrix develops during infancy and occurs on the back of the scalp, nape of the neck, or the entire scalp.

Trichoscopy reveals elliptical nodes of normal hair thickness and intermittent constrictions (defect), internodes at which the hair easily breaks.

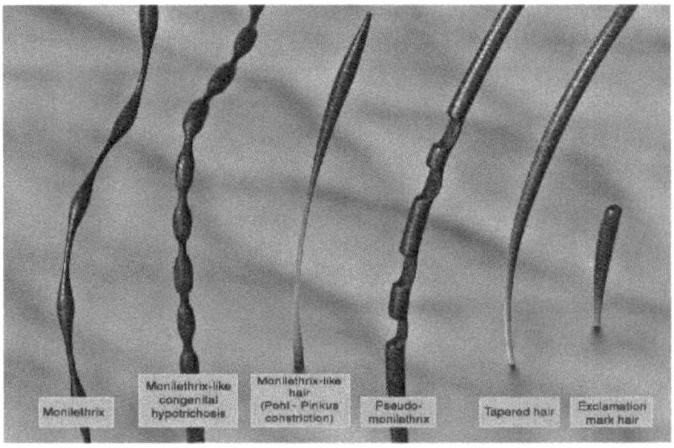

Differential diagnosis:

- Pseudo-monilethrix
- Congenital alopecia
- Trichorrhexis invaginata
- Ectodermal dysplasia

Clinical features of monilethrix:

(a) Typical moniliform hairs with elliptical nodes regularly separated by constricted internodes.

(b) short, sparse hairs, stubble, and follicular papules on the scalp of a young girl with autosomal recessive monilethrix due to *DSG4* mutations.

SchweizerJ, LangbeinL, Rogers MA, Winter H (2007) Exp Cell Res213:2010-2020

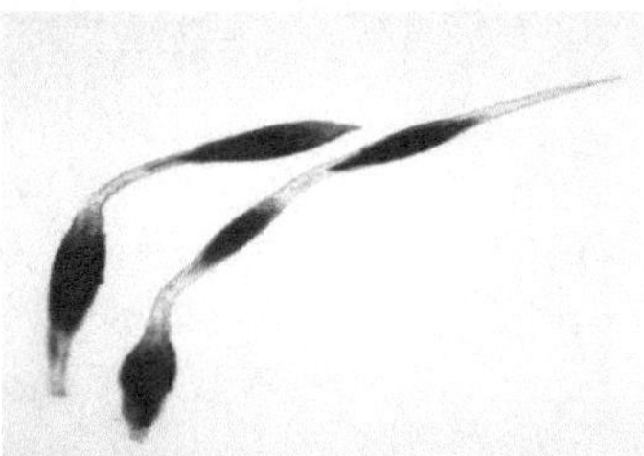

b

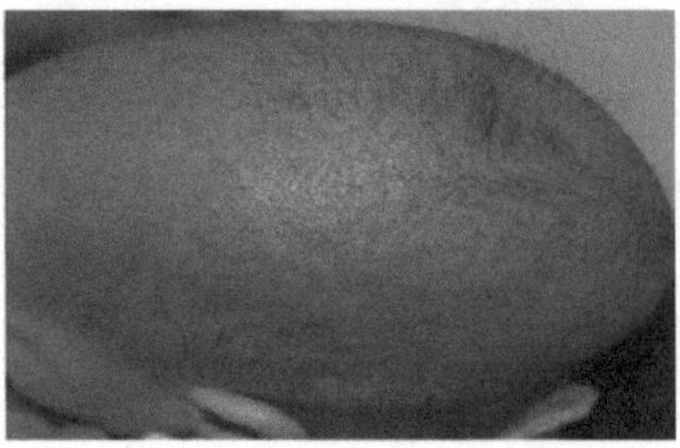

2) **Pili Torti:** (known as twisted hairs)

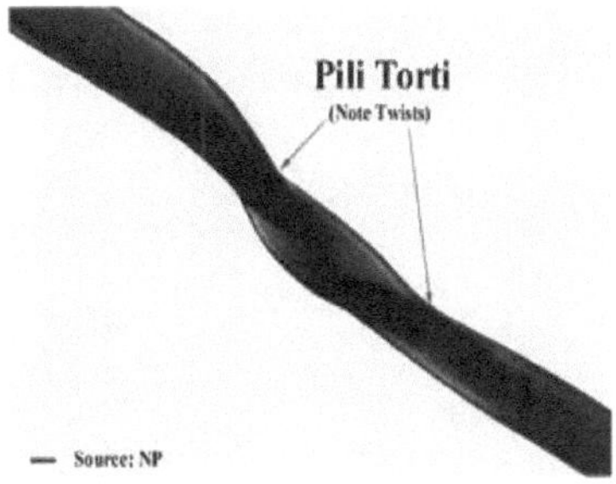

- At an early age of onset, characterized by short and brittle hairs, spangled, easily broken hair at different levels, then the scalp hair after puberty becomes coarse, stiff.
- Mostly flattened hair rotates at angles of 90º, 180º, 360º around its longitudinal axis when viewed through a microscope and trichoscope.
- Non-specific symptoms are associated with many types of hair loss, both inherited and acquired.

Case- 63

A 12-year- old girl presented with difficult hair combing and arrested hair growth. trichoscopic findings: pili torti (white arrows).

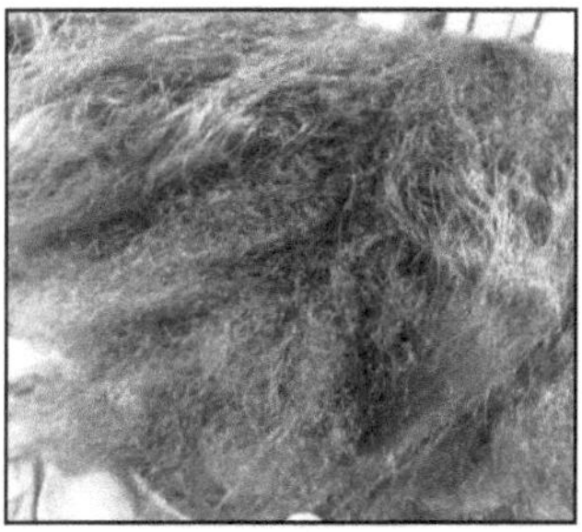
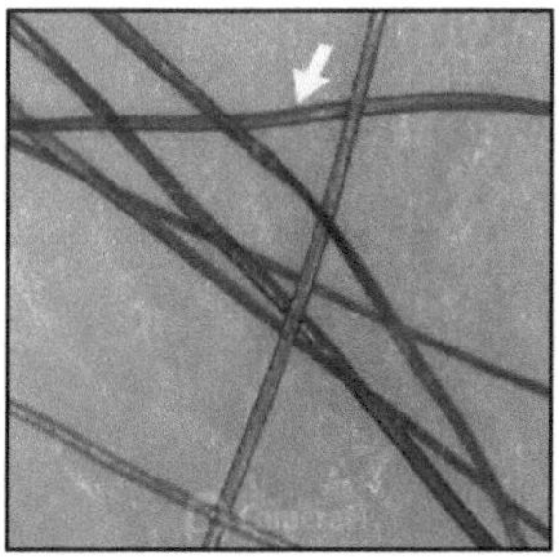
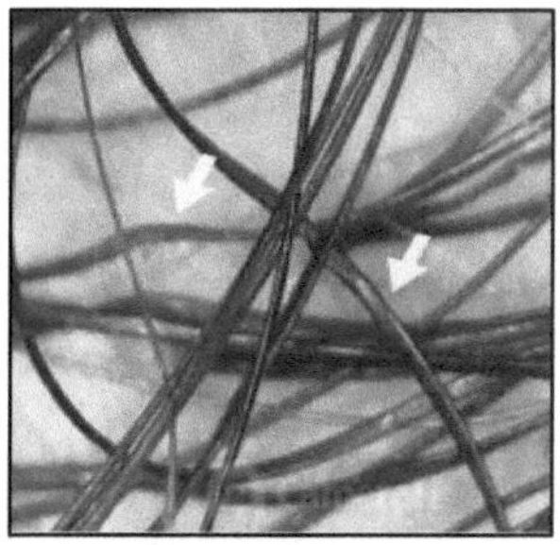

3) **Trichothiodystrophy: (TTD)**

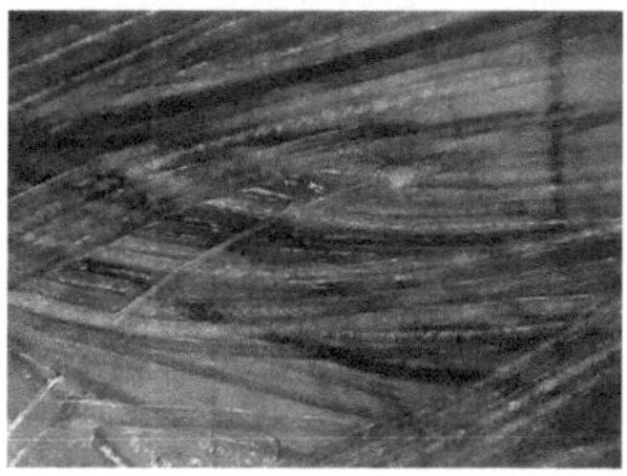

- Characterized by low sulfur or cysteine levels in the hair.
- Varying degrees of clinical presentations from isolated hair shaft abnormality to a more severe developmental delay, intellectual disability, and recurrent infections.
- Trichoscopy does not allow visualization of the most specific feature of trichothiodystrophy: the tiger tail bands.
- Light microscopy(a) will show trichoschisis (transverse fracture through the hair shaft) with or without trichorrhexis nodosa.
- Polarized light(b): Alternating light and dark bands in the hair (tiger tail-like) are visible.

- Both trichoschisis and alternating light and dark bands (tiger tail) are visible under polarized light.

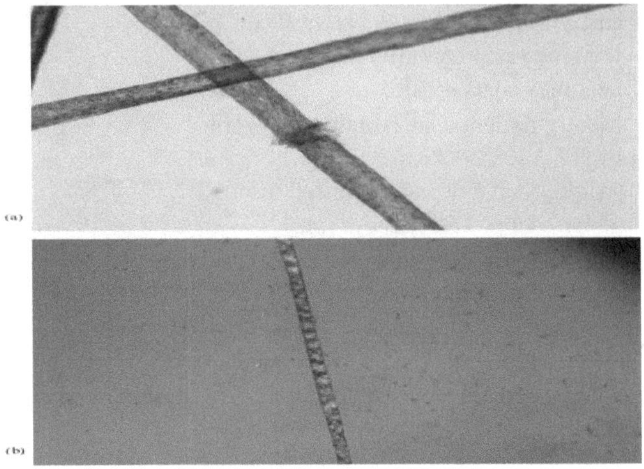

4) **Trichorrexis Invaginata:** (bamboo, matchstick, and golf–tee hairs)
   - It is a ballooning deformity of the hair shaft, also known as bamboo hair (regularly bended ribbon sign).
   - On a handheld dermoscope, it appears as multiple small nodules spaced along the shaft.
   - High magnifications produced by videodermoscope show invagination of the distal portion of the hair shaft into its proximal portion, forming a ball-in-cup appearance.
   - It is a specific anomaly considered a marker for Netherton syndrome, which is an AR genodermatosis observed more frequently in females. Characteristic features could be visualized within the eyebrows.

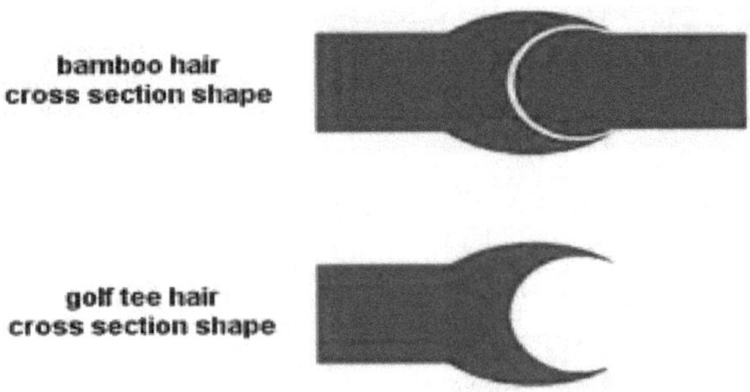

Case- 64

A 13-year- old girl presented with generalized eczematous itchy skin her diagnosis Netherton syndrome was made on the physical examination findings presence of double edge scales of ichthyosis linearis circumflex and associated hair shaft finding (trichorrhexis invaginata), which confirmed by microscopic examination.

The expanded proximal end of an invaginate node after break has occurred while the distal hair end has concave cupped appearance.

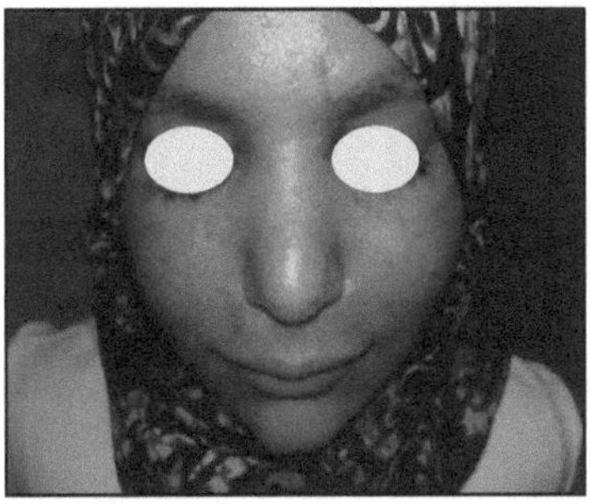

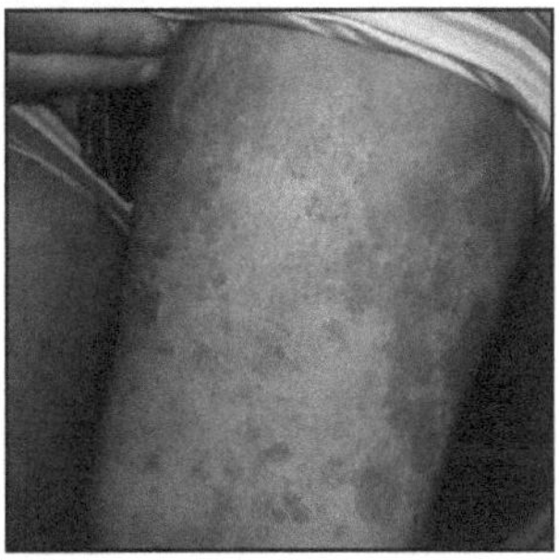

(a) Short broken eyebrows

(b) Ichthyosis linearis circumflexa showing squamous double borders.

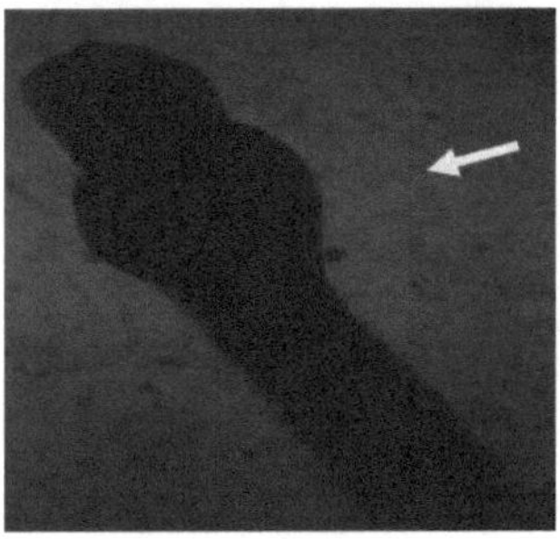

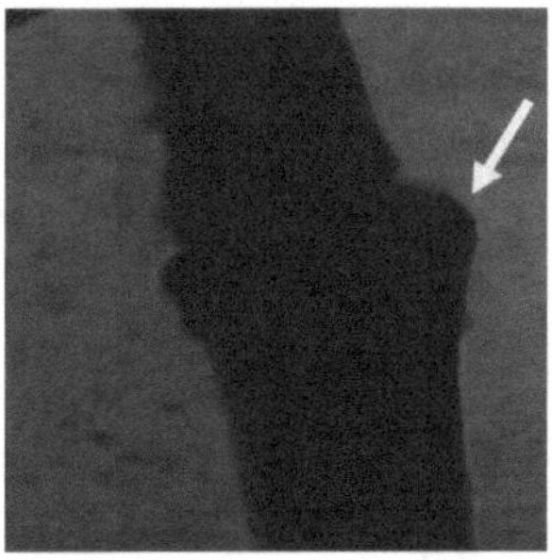

The distal hair shaft is telescoped into the proximal hair shaft (white arrow), forming a ball-and-socket appearance.

Note:

Other hair anomalies may manifest as: Pilitorti and Trichorrhexis nodosa.

The differential diagnosis:

- Atopic dermatitis.
- Generalized seborrheic dermatitis.
- Psoriasis.

5) Trichorrhexis nodosa: TN

It is defined as the presence of nodules of fracture on the hair shafts. It may be acquired in patients with normal hair through exposure to a sufficient level of trauma.

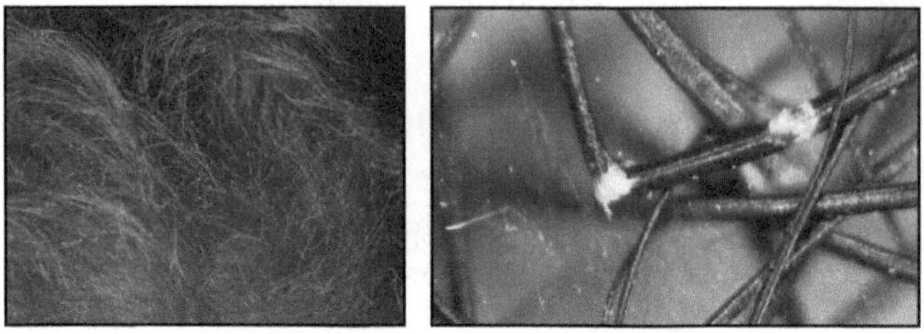

Trichoscopy using videodermoscopy shows thrust paint brushes as if two brushes are thrust into each other (Non-polarized mode, 70x magnification; fotofinder, Germany).

Clinically appears as hair nodules-Health Jade team.

Proximal TN (red arrows) in an alopecia patient:

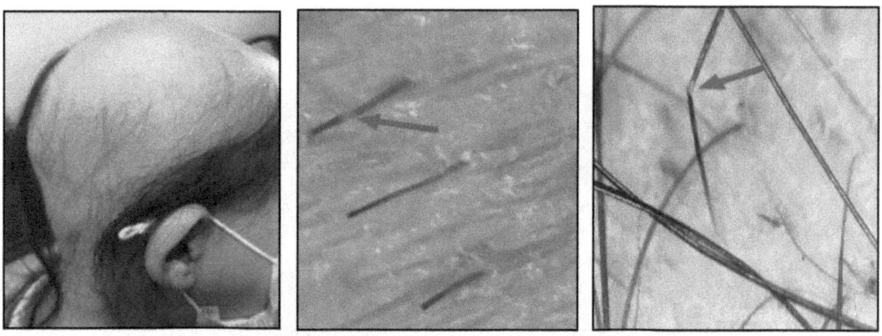

Proximal TN (red arrows) in a trichotellomania patient:

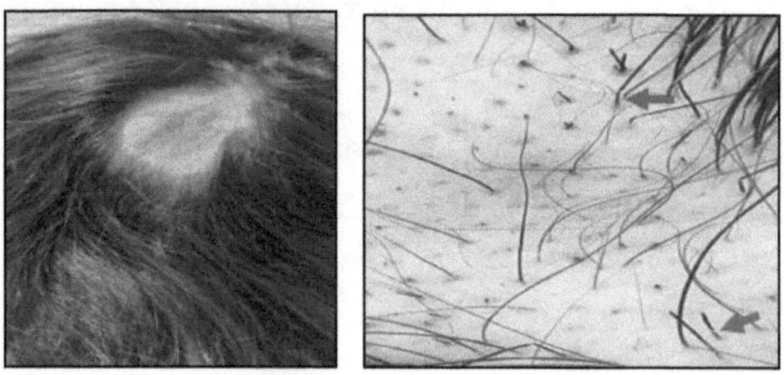

6) Pili Trianguli and Canaliculi= uncombable hair syndrome:

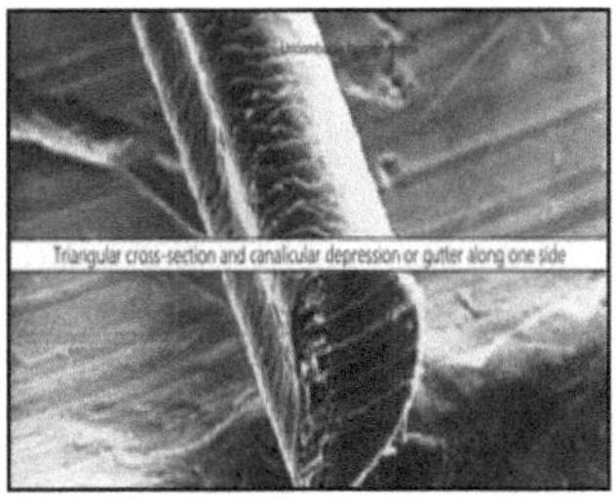

- As dry, blond, shiny hair, flat, thinner, curly, twisted.
- Spun glass hair, elliptical or oval in cross-section.
- Longitudinal grooves make hair rigid.
- Due to abnormal keratinization of the inner root sheath.
- Some cases improve spontaneously in childhood.
- Some hairs may have trichorrhexis nodes.

Case- 65

A 28-year-old man presents a dry, wrinkled hair difficult to comb since birth.

Trichoscopic findings: Flat hair with longitudinal groove (blue arrow).

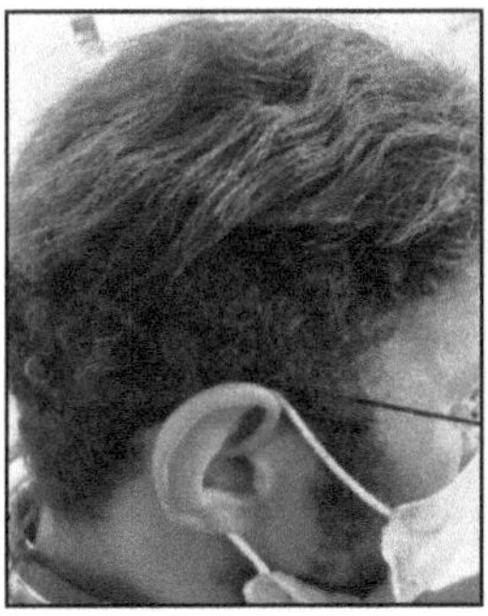

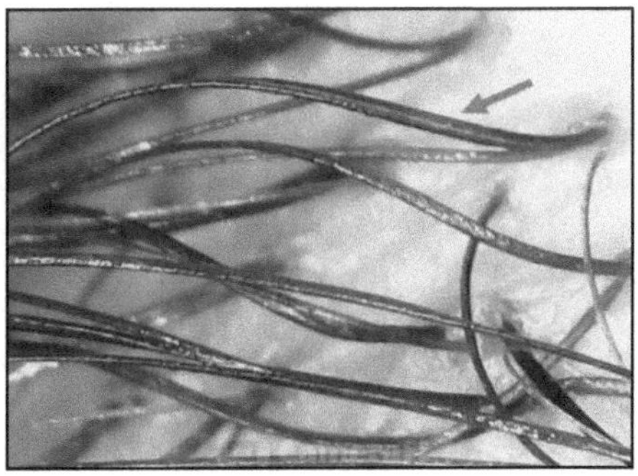

7) Trichoclasis:

Clean transverse fracture across the hair shaft with defect in cuticle, it may be secondary to conditions that weaken the hair, while trichoschisis is similar to trichoclasis but with intact cuticle. Some authors use the terms trichoschisis and trichoclasia interchangeably.

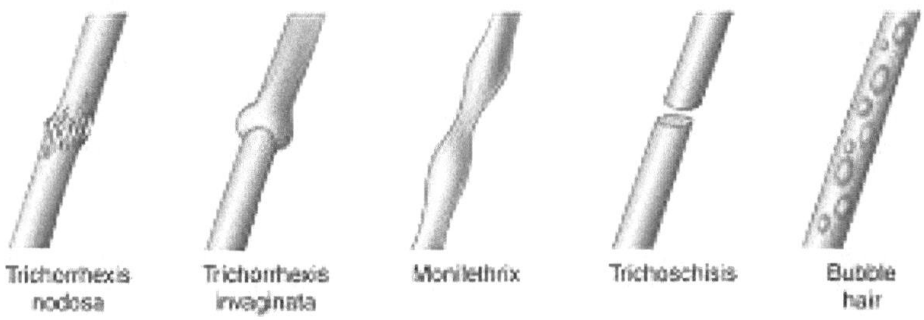

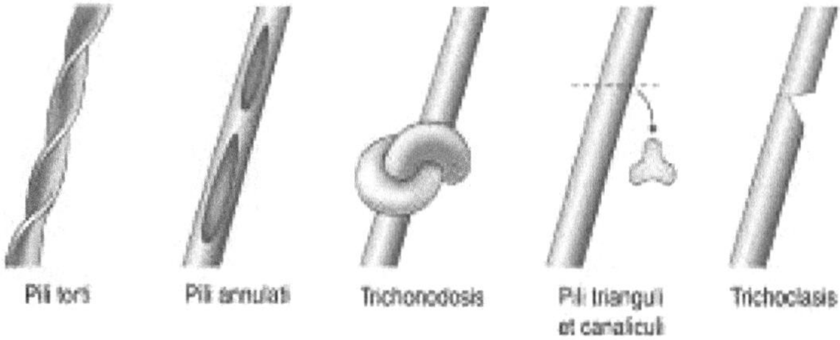

8) **Pili bifurcates:**
The hair shaft bifurcates into two parts and is covered by its own cuticle; the parts may rejoin distally (white arrow).

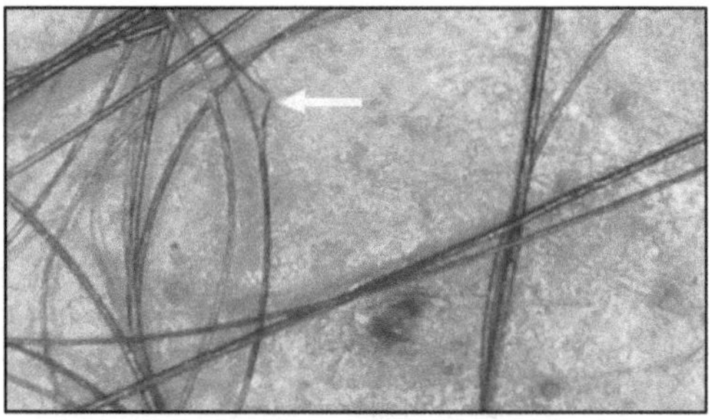

9) **Pili multigemini:**
- Formed by a cluster of short hair shafts emerging from one hair follicle, the hair shafts are surrounded by a common outer root sheath, but each hair has its own root sheath.
- Hyperpigmented papules with short and irregular hairs; common sites: the beard of men and the scalp of children.

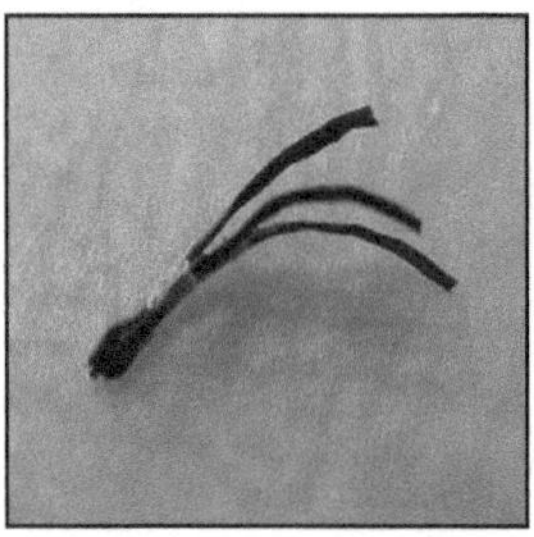

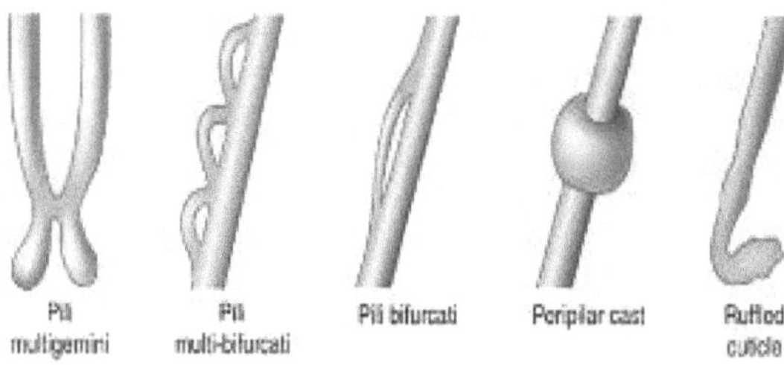

Hair shaft disorders without hair fragility

Pili Annulati:

- Usually, the hair appears shiny and banded (light& dark), due to air-filled spaces between the macrofibrillar units of the hair cortex.
- Trichoscopy features include bright bands caused by light scattered from clusters of air-filled cavities in the hair.
- Air space in the cortex appears darker in light microscopy.

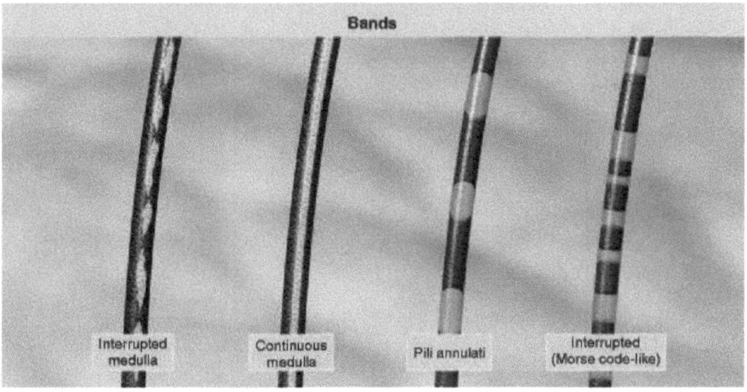

Woolly hair syndrome (WHS):
A group of hair shaft disorders characterized by short, kinked, tightly curled hair, traditionally diagnosed by clinical examination and light microscopy.
Trichoscopy allowed to differentiate between healthy curly hair and the WHS hair shafts demonstrated a crawling snake appearance with short wave cycles.

Case- 66

Two sisters of non –consanguineous parents aged 1.5 and 11 year with sparse dry sticky difficult combing and lighter in color and did not grow long, there were no nails and dental or other skin changes. Laboratory investigations were normal.
Light microscopy and trichoscopy showed: crawling snake kinking hair shaft 180 degree along it is axis and monilethrix like hair and trichorrhexis nodosa.
Scanning electron microscopy was not performed as it was not available in the clinic.
Trichoscopic findings:
Woolly hair; kinking hair shaft (red arrow) and monilethrix like hair (yellow arrow), trichorrhexis nodosa (blue arrow), crawling snake appearance (white arrow).

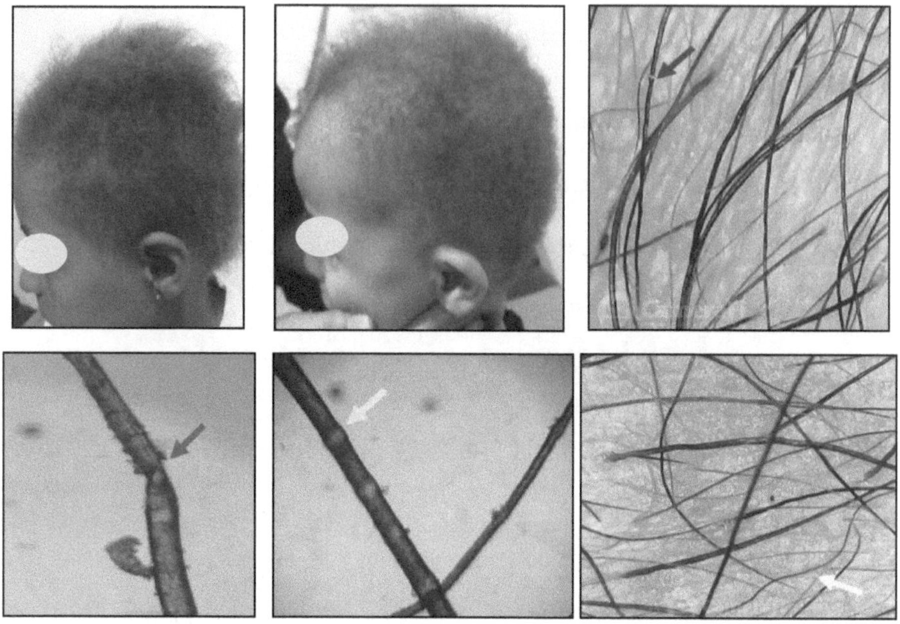

7. Hair Damage:

Trichorrhexis Nodosa:
Broken hairs with nodes along the hair shaft, mentioned above.

Trichoptilosis:
Refer to the splitting or fraying of the distal hair shaft, which occurs due to damage or tearing away of the cuticle layer, mentioned above.

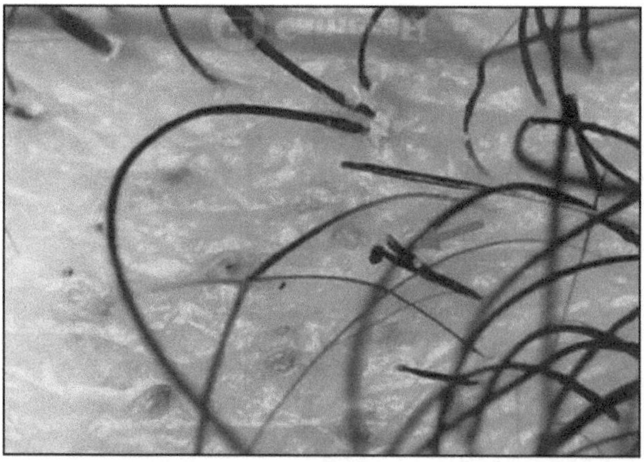

Broom hair in non-cicatricial alopecia

Multiple short full-thickness hairs emerging from one follicular unit in a brush–like pattern can differentiate pili multigemini from compound follicles (Red arrow).

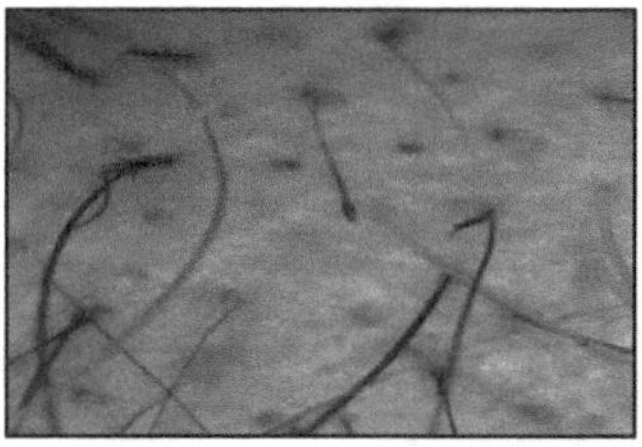

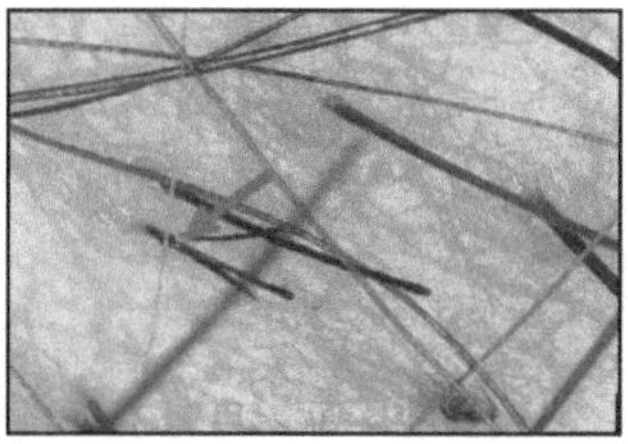

Bubble hair:

Deformed hair shafts due to heat exposure caused by dryers and curling irons.

Bubble hair: dermoscopy shows bubbles appearing as white oval spaces with Swiss-cheese structure *(FotoFinder: System GmbH, Bad Birnach, Germany, original magnification: 370.)*

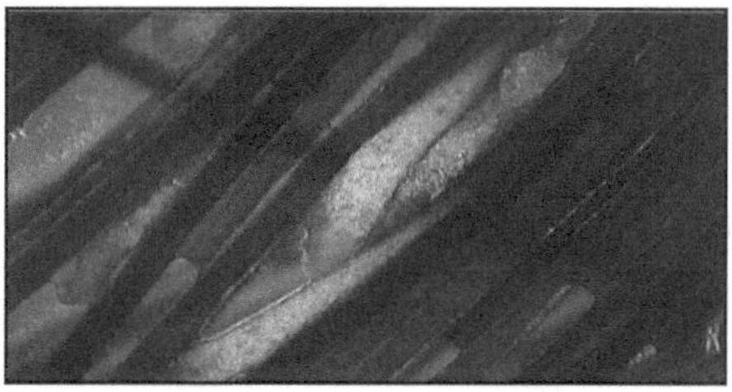

Trichonodosis (hair knotting):

- It is an acquired, transient condition in which a single (blue arrow) or double knot (white arrow) occurs in the hair shaft, either spontaneously or in response to scratching.
- It is observed in a patient with short, curly hair.
- Usually, an incidental finding of little clinical significance.

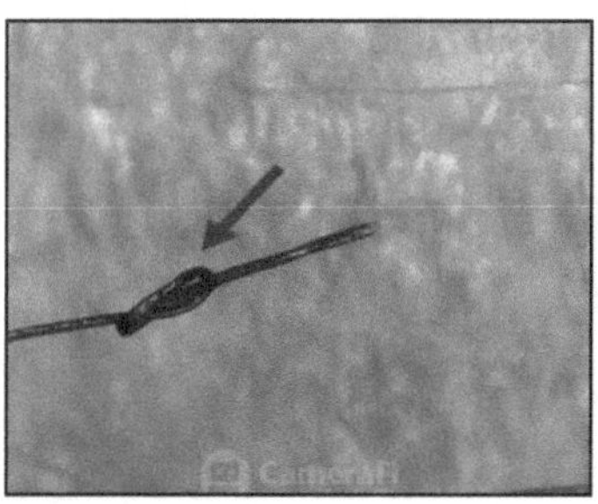

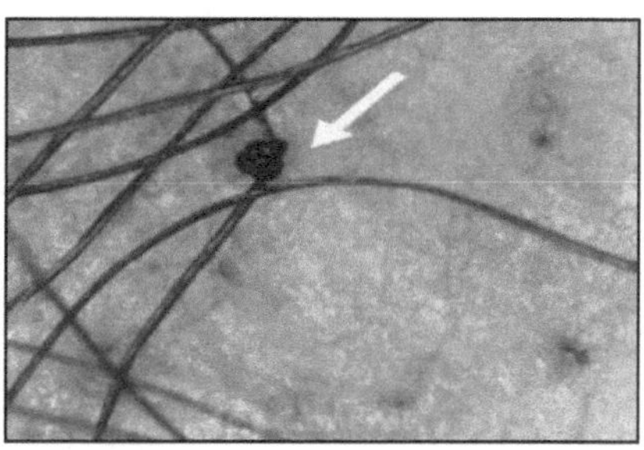

Acute hair matting: (also called Plica polonica and bird's nest hair)

A rare, acquired condition that presents as a sudden solid mass of permanent matting of scalp hair on the vertex in otherwise healthy individuals. Hair twists irregularly and is severely entangled, forming a stiff, tightly packed mass of keratin over the head, cemented together with dirt and exudates.

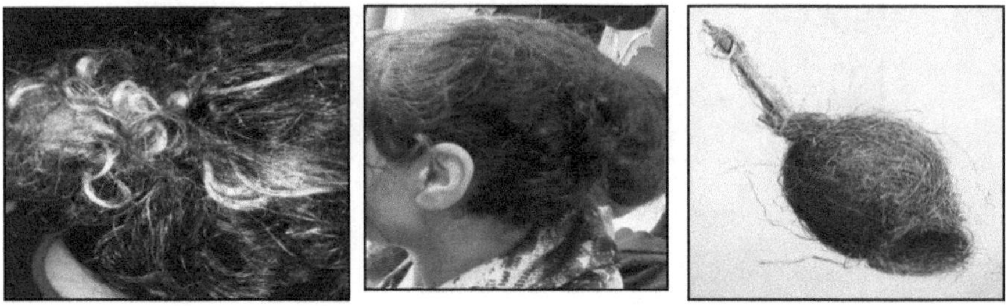

Photos for plica polonica: Female patients had a similar history of sudden onset of difficult hair combing- bird's nest-like.

Camouflage products: to cover alopecia

1) **Powders:**

Male patient applying dark powder to cover alopecia areata on the scalp.

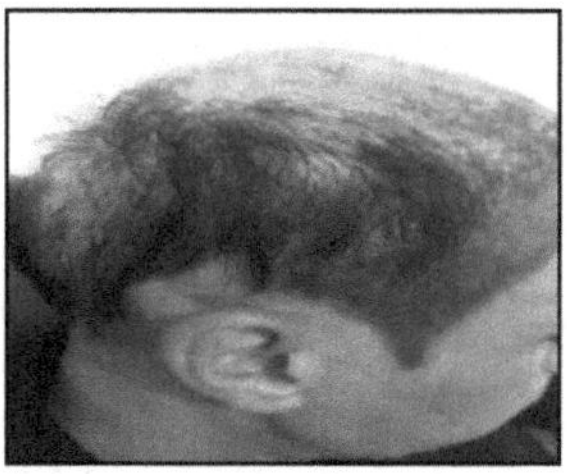

2) **Fibers**

Different dyes create different shades of keratin fibers that can match any natural hair color.

Keratin fibers result in thick-looking hair. This occurs due to the natural positive static hair follicles that attract and stick a negative charge on keratin fibers.

Clinical photo for female patient 37yr old presents patchy alopecia applying keratin fibers; toppik (white arrow), which may be misinterpretation as broken hairs.

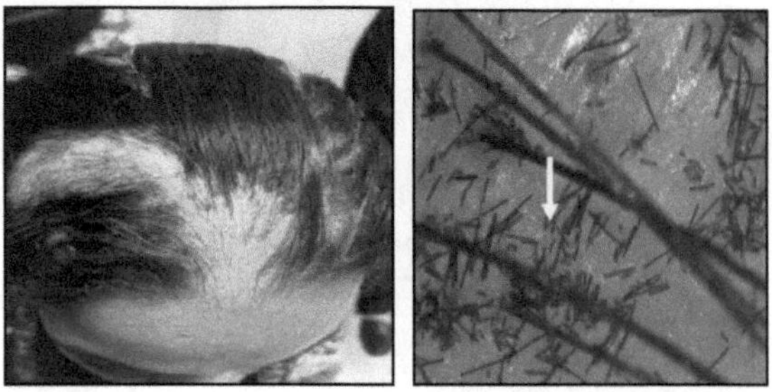

3) Tattoos

Scalp micropigmentation (SMP) is a tattoo technique where tattoo pigments are placed on the scalp in a stippling pattern to look like a shaved head of hair.
4-Medications: Dithranol ointment, penetrates and stains the follicular opening, may be seen as black dots.

8. Infections

8.1 Tinea capitus:

- Cutaneous fungal infection or dermatophytosis of the scalp that occurs mainly in children.
- Mainly caused by microsporum and trichophyton species.
- Clinically is characterized by the presence of hair loss areas with coexistent scaling, inflammation, or pustules.
- Diagnosis is confirmed by fungus visualization through direct mycological exam or growth of the specific fungus in a suitable culture environment.
- The presence of characteristic trichoscopic features of tinea capitus is sufficient to establish the initial diagnosis and introduce treatment before culture results are available.

Comma hair:

- It is a short, curved C-shaped, like a comma, and is homogenous in pigmentation and thickness; it is seen in both endothrix and ecthothrix infections.
- Bending of the infected hair shafts and formation of comma hairs probably are a result of partial damage to hair shafts filled with hyphae or damage to the hair cuticle.
- Question mark: comma-shaped modified hair.
- Occasionally detected in patients with alopecia areata and trichotillomania.

Corkscrew:

- Presence of multiple hair twists and an intensely coiled shape
- Spiral-like hair is seen in both ecthotrix, endothrix TC
- Mostly formed by dermatophytes of the genera (Trichophyton and Microsporum).

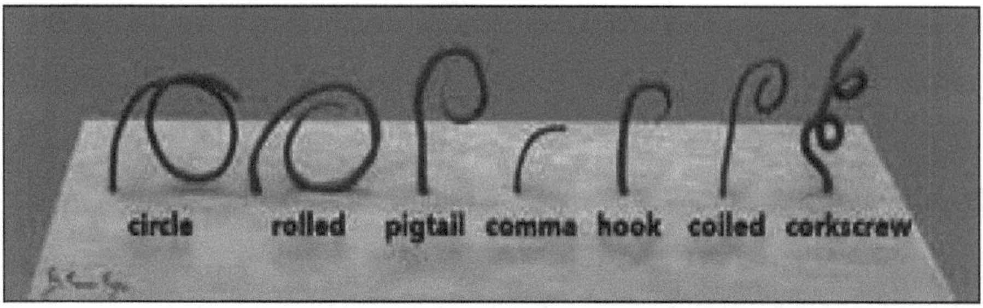

Schematic illustration of the forms of circular hair and variations,

Case- 67

A3-year- girl presents with small scaly patches scattered on vertex for one year.

Trichoscopic findings: Corkscrew hair (black arrow), comma hair (red arrow), and horseshoe hair (blue arrow).

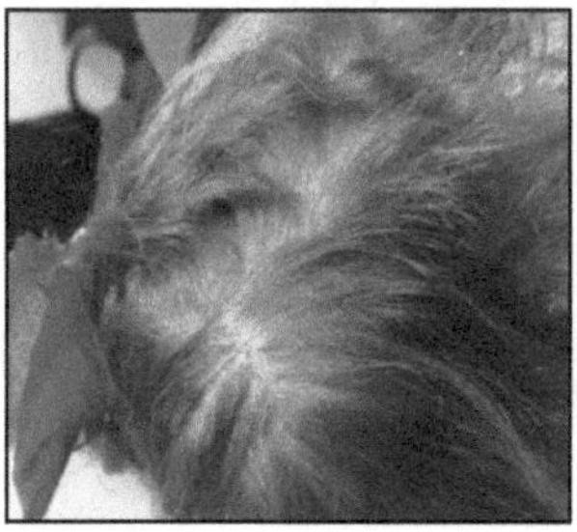

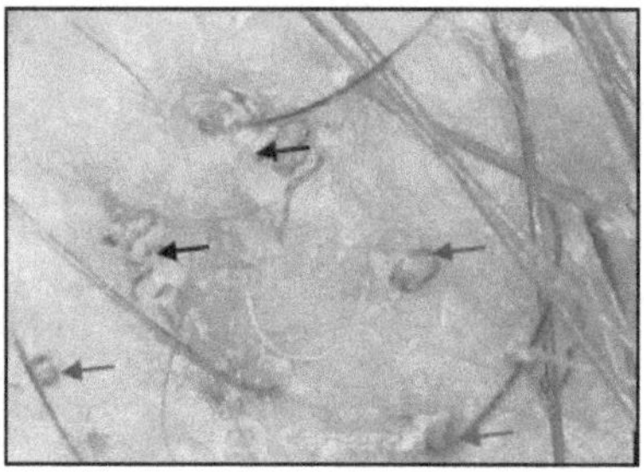

Z hair:

It is zigzag hair with multiple bends as a result of an incomplete transverse fracture along the hair shaft.

Morse code: also called bar code (transverse bands)

- Short, interrupted gaps in the hair shafts.
- Difficult to distinguish from trichorrexis nodosa on trichoscopy with immersion fluid.
- On dry trichoscopy, tinea capitus bands are transparent, whereas trichorrhexis nodosa appears white.

Case- 68

An 8-year- boy presented with large scaly patch of hair loss on occipital region.

Trichoscopic findings:

- Before cleaned with alcohol swab- morse code (yellow arrow).
- After cleaned with alcohol swab-comma shape (blue arrow), black dot (red arrow), bent hair (green arrow), and z hair (white arrow).

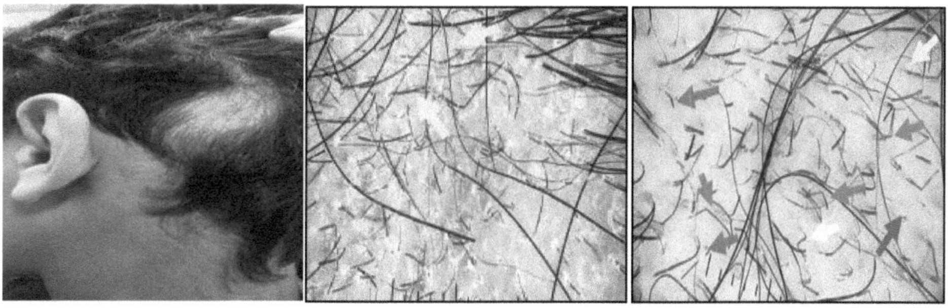

Note:
About Zigzag hairs
- Resulting from trichorrhexis nodosa may be observed on the early acute phase of alopecia areata.
- Described only in patient with ectothrix type of fungal infection.

Case- 69

A12-year- boy presenting with a single scaly patch of hair loss on frontal scalp for one month.

Trichoscopic findings: comma hair (blue arrow), corkscrew (red arrow), U-shaped hair (green arrow), and bent hair (yellow arrow).

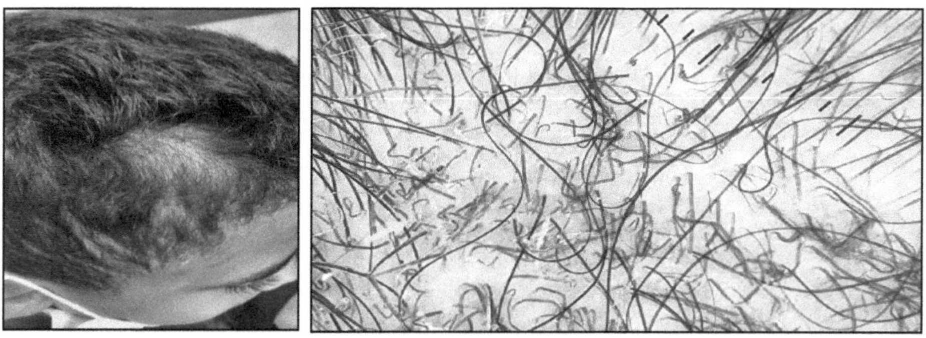

Note:

- **i-hair:** There may be hypopigmented band (gap) directly beneath the dark distal end, making these hairs looks like the letter i.
- Hair changes are not specific in TC
- Broken hairs, black dots, perifollicular and diffuse scaling are commonly observed in tinea capitis.

Block hair:

They are very short with a transverse horizontal distal end (red arrows).

Bent hair: also called elbow hair

They are characterized by bending of the hair shaft with homogeneous thickness and pigmentation, in contrast to comma hairs, with no hair shaft shortening. They were only observed in patients with ectothrix-type fungal infection.

Tinea capitus on trichoscopy presents multiple block hair (red arrows), bent hair (blue arrow), Morse code (yellow arrow).

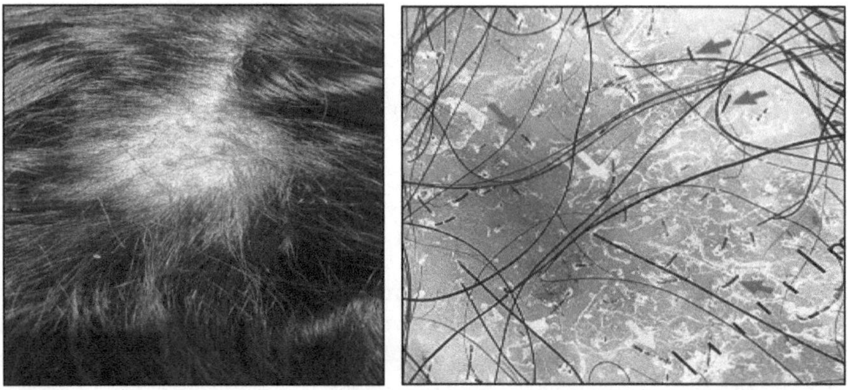

Horseshoe hair: U-shaped

Trichoscopy of tinea capitus: comma hairs are the most common specific Findings.
Dr. Donovans' articles, April 6, 2022

Findings	Prevalence
Comma Hairs	52%
Corkscrew Hairs	32%
Morse Code Hairs	22%
Zigzag Hairs	21%
Bent Hairs	27%
Black dots	10%
i Hairs	10%

8.2 Piedra

Piedra is a Spanish word that means stone.

Black piedra: Also known as trichomycosis nodosa, tinea nodosa, or trichosporosis, is piedra hortae fungal infection of the hair shafts resulting in the formation of small black firm nodules. The scalp most common site of involvement. Trichoscopic examination: It shows multiple oval or elongate-shaped nodules

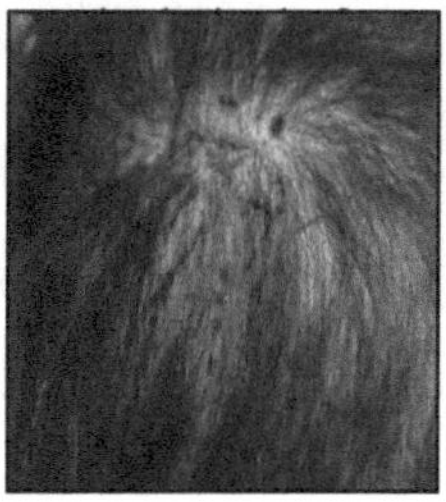

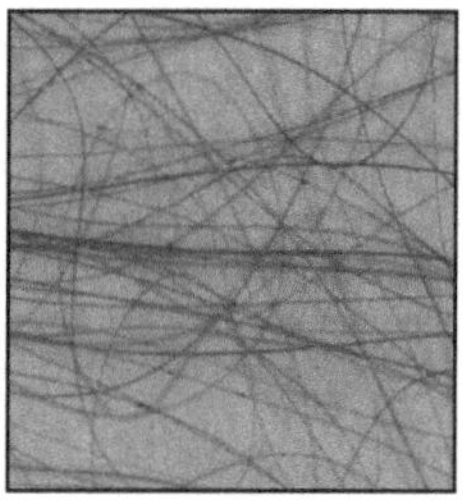

White piedra: (trihosporon beigelii fungus)

- They are fusiform, soft in consistency, white or light brown, loosely adherent, mainly attached to the distal portion of the hair.
- The scalp most common site of involvement, but the beard and pubic areas may be affected.
- Trichoscopy of white piedra showing oval whitish masses along the hair shafts.

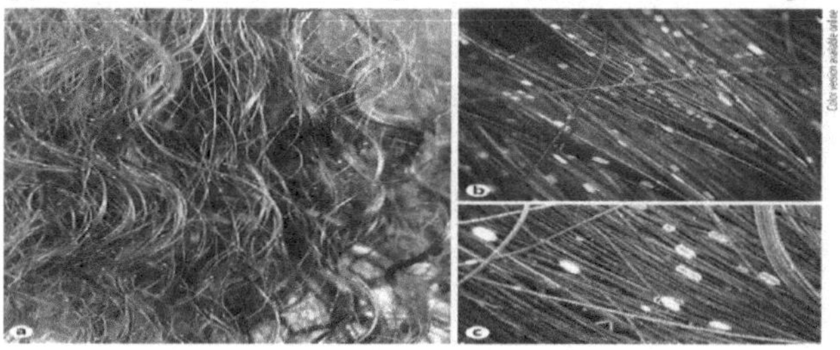

9. Infestations:

Pediculosis: refers to lice infestation of any part of the body

- Three varieties are: Pediculosis humanus capitus (head louse), Pthirus pubis (crab louse), and Pediculus corporis (body louse).
- Head-lice infestation is the most frequent in school-age children.
- Head lice are spread through direct head-to-head contact with an infected person.
- Each egg or nit may hatch one nymph that will grow and develop into an adult louse.

Case- 70

A 7-year-girl complaining of sever scalp itching on physical examination she has profuse scalp nits .

Trichoscopy demonstration of a viable nits containing nymphs appear as dark brown pyriform-shaped structures attached to the shaft (yellow arrows).

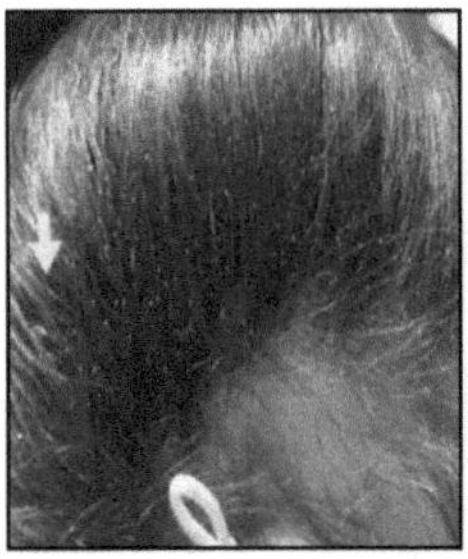

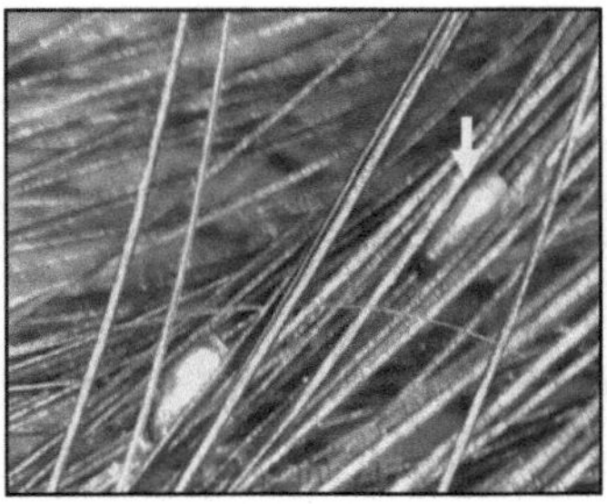

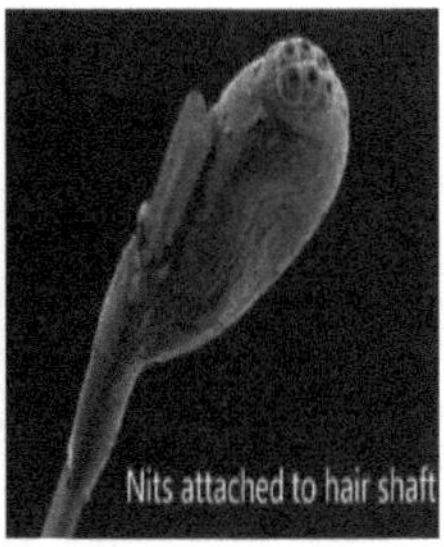

Case- 71

Boy 2years-old his mother complaint that sever itching disturbed her baby sleep.

On examination with contact non polarizing handheld dermoscope shows brown nits on eye lashes, sticky and clumpy eye lashes .

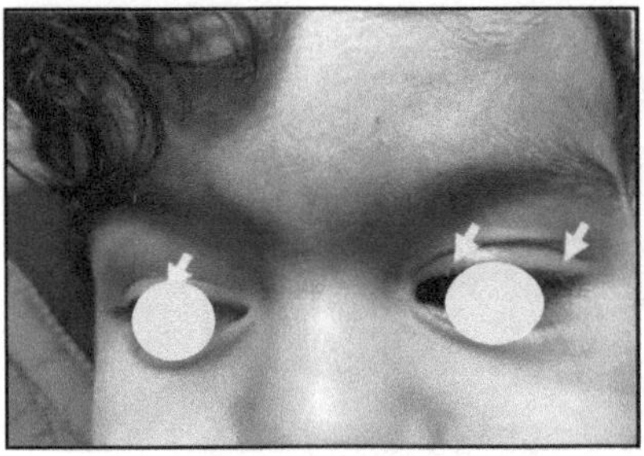

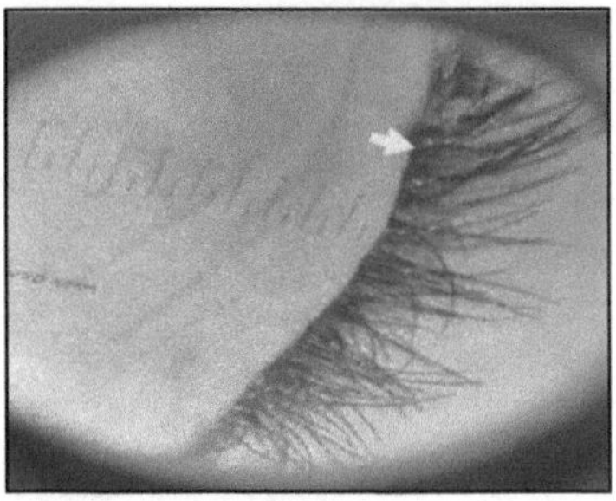

Phthiriasis palpebrarum (eyelash lice) is a rare type of eyelid infestation caused by phthiriasis pubis, commonly known as crab lice, sometimes misdiagnosed as blepharitis of the eyelid.

Causes of nodules on the hair shaft:

- Black piedra
- White piedra
- Nits
- Hair cast: elongated tubular structures encircling the hair shaft and easily movable along it.
- Trichomycosis
- Trichorrhexis nodosa

References:

1. Saitoh M, Uzuka M, Sakamoto M. Human hair cycle. J Invest Dermatol 1970.
2. Saraogi P, Dhurat R. Automated digital image analysis (Trichoscan) for human hair growth analysis: ease versus errors. Int J Trich 2010.
3. Ross EK, Vincenzi C, Tosti A. Videodermoscopy in the evaluation of hair and scalp disorders. J Am Acad Dermatol. 2006.
4. Kim GW, Jung HJ, Ko HC, Kim MB, Lee WJ, Lee SJ, et al. Dermoscopy can be useful in differentiating scalp psoriasis from seborrheic dermatitis. Br J Dermatol. 2011.
5. Overnight Alopecia: A Subtype of Acute Diffuse and Total Alopecia? Int J Trichology . 2019 Jul-Aug.
6. Masahiro Fukuyama , Misaki Kinoshita-Ise , Yohei Sato, Manabu Ohyama . Elucidation of demographic, clinical, and trichoscopic features for early diagnosis of self-healing acute diffuse and total alopecia. J Dermatol. 2020 Jun.
7. Ali Abdulghani Ramadan & Hindav Mirdan Khaleel trichoscopic comparison between telogen effluvium and androgenic alopecia vol 17 no 1 (2023): Duhok Medical Journal.
8. Deren Özcan.Pediatric androgenetic alopecia: a retrospective review of clinical characteristics, hormonal assays, and metabolic syndrome risk factors in 23 patients. Anais Brasileiros de Dermatologia, Volume 97, Issue 2, March–April 2022, Pages 166-172
9-Zaballos P, Serrano P, Flores G, Bañuls J, Thomas L, Llambrich A, et al. Dermoscopy of tumours arising in naevus sebaceous: a morphological study of 58 cases. J Eur Acad Dermatol Venereol. 2015.
10. Cribier B, Scrivener Y, Grosshans E. Tumors arising in nevus sebaceus: a study of 596 cases. J Am Acad Dermatol. 2000.
11. Brooke RC, Griffiths CE. Folliculitis decalvans. Clin Exp Dermatol. 2001.
12. Perkins W. Acne keloidalis nuchae. In: *Treatment of skin disease: comprehensive therapeutic strategies.* 4th edn: Elsevier Limited, 2014
13. Ahmed Sadek, Trichoscopy of generalised noncicatricial hair loss, DermNet content department, May 2022.
14. Osama Moawad, Broken Hair Ends and Hair Shaft Abnormalities, 18, 2020 Vivien Chen , Lauren Strazzulla , Sara M Asbeck , Fernanda Bellodi Schmidt . Etiology, management, and outcomes of pediatric telogen effluvium: A single-center study in the United States. Pediatr Dermatol. 2023 Jan.
15. Inui S, Nakajima T, Itami S. Temporal triangular alopecia: trichoscopic diagnosis. J Dermatol. 2012.
16. Dlova NC, Jordaan FH, Sarig O, Sprecher E. Autosomal dominant inheritance of central centrifugal cicatricial alopecia in black South Africans. J Am Acad Dermatol 2014.
17-Anna Waśkiel-Burnat, Adriana Rakowska, Mariusz Sikora, Piotr Ciechanowicz, Małgorzata Olszewska, and Lidia Rudnicka Trichoscopy of Tinea Capitis:A Systemic Review Dermatol Ther (Heidelb). 2020.

18. Gupta AK, Mays RR, Versteeg SG, et al. Tinea capitis in children: a systematic review of management. J Eur Acad Dermatol Venereol. 2018.
19-Tosti A, Lorizzo M, Piraccini BM, Androgenetic alopecia in children: report of 20 cases. Br J Dermatol. 2006.
20. Melike Kibar, Şebnem Aktan,1 and Muzaffer Bilgin2 Dermoscopic Findings in Scalp Psoriasis and Seborrheic Dermatitis; Two New Signs; Signet Ring Vessel and Hidden HairIndian J Dermatol. 2015 Jan-Feb.
21. Anna Waśkiel-Burnat, Joanna Czuwara, Leszek Blicharz, Małgorzata Olszewska, Lidia RudnickaDifferential diagnosis of red scalp. The importance of trichoscopy*Clinical and Experimental Dermatology* llad366, 03 November 2023.
22. Neelam R, Nakamura M, Tejasvi T. Dermoscopy of aplasia cutis congenita: a case report and review of the literature. Dermatol. 2021;11(1): e2021154.
23. Azhar Ahmed. Hind Almohanna. Jacob Griggs. Antonella TostGenetic Hair Disorders: A ReviewDermatol Ther (Heidelb) https://doi.org/10.1007/s13555-019-0313-2
24.Giulia Liberati M.D., Michela Starace M.D., Annalisa Patrizi M.D., Bianca Maria Piraccini M.D., Ph.D.Neonatal Alopecia Due to Birth Trauma: Case Report and Trichoscopic Findings First published: 31 May 2016
25-Alexandro Bonifaz , Andrés Tirado-Sánchez , Javier Araiza , Alejandra Rodríguez-Leviz , Daniela Guzmán-Sánchez , Selene Gutiérrez-Mendoza , Laura Castrejón White Piedra: Clinical, Mycological, and Therapeutic Experience of Fourteen Cases Skin Appendage Disorder. 2019 Apr.
26. Feroze Kaliyadan, Joel Kuruvilla, Heba Yousef Al Ojail, and Sayed A Quadri. Clinical and Dermoscopic Study of Pseudofolliculitis of the Beard Area Int J Trichology. 2016 Jan-Mar.
27. Melike Kibar, Şebnem Aktan,1 and Muzaffer Bilgin2 Dermoscopic Findings in Scalp Psoriasis and Seborrheic Dermatitis; Two New Signs; Signet Ring Vessel and Hidden Hair, Indian J Dermatol. 2015 Jan-Feb.
28. A. Giacaman , a, J. Ferrando b [Translated article] Keys to the Diagnosis of Hair Shaft Disorders: Part IClaves diagnósticas en displasias pilosas I Volume 113, Issue 2, February 2022,
29. Pham CM, Krejci-Manwaring J. Loose anagen hair syndrome: An underdiagnosed condition in males. Pediatr Dermatol 2010.
30. Na Wu, Hong Zhang, Feng Yuan Sun Phthiriasis palpebrarum: A case of eyelash infestation with Pthirus pubis, Experimental and Therapeutic Medicine; March 6, 2017.
31. Sperling LC, DiGiovanna JJ. "Curly" wood and tiger tails: an explanation for light and dark banding with polarization in trichothiodystrophy. Arch Dermatol. 2003.

32.Rudnicka, Lidia; Olszewska, Małgorzata; Waśkiel, Anna; Rakowska, Adriana (2018). "Trichoscopy in Hair Shaft Disorders". Dermatologic Clinics. 36 (4). Elsevier BV: 421–430. doi:10.1016/j.det.2018.05.009. ISSN 0733-8635.
33. Ben Abdelghani K, Mahmoud I, Chatelus E, Sordet C, Gottenberg JE, Sibilia J. Multicentric reticulohistiocytosis: an autoimmune systemic disease? Case report of an association with erosive rheumatoid arthritis and systemic Sjogren syndrome. Joint Bone Spine. 2010.
34. Tosti A, Torres F, Misciali C, Vincenzi C, Starace M, Miteva M, Romanelli P. Follicular red dots: a novel dermoscopic pattern observed in scalp discoid lupus erythematosus. Arch Dermatol. 2009.
35. Sharma P, Nassereddin A, Sonthalia S. Black Piedra. [Updated 2020 Aug 10]. In: StatPearls. Treasure Island (FL): StatPearls Publishing; 2020 Jan-. Available from: https://www.ncbi.nlm.nih.gov/books/NBK545178.
36. J. Romer. R. Grimalt Trichoscopy: Essentials for the dermatologist, published May 2015.

FSC
www.fsc.org
MIX
Papier | Fördert
gute Waldnutzung
FSC® C083411

Kolibri 360 GmbH
Ferdinand-Jühlke-Straße 7
99095 Erfurt, Deutschland
produktsicherheit@kolibri360.de

Druck:
CPI Druckdienstleistungen GmbH
im Auftrag der
Kolibri 360 GmbH
Ferdinand-Jühlke-Str. 7
99095 Erfurt